Reforming the
Health Care Market

An Interpretive
Economic History

Reforming the Health Care Market

An Interpretive Economic History

David F. Drake

GEORGETOWN UNIVERSITY PRESS / WASHINGTON, D.C.

Georgetown University Press, Washington, D.C.
© 1994 by Georgetown University Press. All rights reserved.
Printed in the United States of America
10 9 8 7 6 5 4 3 2 1   1994
THIS VOLUME IS PRINTED ON ACID-FREE OFFSET BOOK PAPER

Library of Congress Cataloging-in-Publication Data

Drake, David F.
    Reforming the health care market : an interpretive economic
history / David F. Drake.
        p.   cm.
        1. Medical economics—United States—History—20th century.
    2. Health care reform—United States.   I. Title.
    RA410.53.D73   1994
    362.1'0973—dc20
    ISBN 0-87840-567-4. — ISBN 0-87840-568-2 (pbk.)   94-13475

To Cy and Alex
with great appreciation

Contents

    1980 to the Present   104
    SHIFTING BALANCE OF HEALTH CARE PROVIDERS 106,
    THE RESURGENCE OF HEALTH INSURERS 114,   PASSIVE HEALTH CARE
    CONSUMERS 121,   STATE OF THE HEALTH CARE MARKETPLACE 127

6   The Retrospective on the Health Care Industry: What
    Went Wrong and Why   129
    OVERINVESTMENT IN SCIENCE AND TECHNOLOGY 130,   WHY DID
    AMERICANS OVERINVEST IN SCIENTIFIC MEDICINE? 143,
    THE PRINCIPAL SOURCE OF MARKET FAILURE 153

7   The Promise of Health Care Reform   157
    THE CLINTON REFORM PROPOSAL 158,   A REFORM PLAN REDRESSING
    PAST MARKET TRANSGRESSIONS 169,   WHAT ELSE CAN BE GAINED
    FROM REFORM 193,   APPENDIX 195

    Chapter Notes   199
    References   207
    Index   217

List of Tables

Preface

This study was started more than 14 years ago when I took a partial leave from the American Hospital Association to prepare an economic history of the hospital industry. During 1980 and 1981 materials were developed on the pre-Medicare history of hospitals, but work on the project stopped in 1982, when I took on the added responsibilities of the association's chief financial officer. After my early retirement in 1992 the project was expanded to encompass the entire health care industry, and full-time work was devoted to completing the study.

The pre-Medicare period was marked by great organizational stability or even rigidity, but much about the health care market had changed during my 10-year absence from the study. At least outwardly the industry had taken on many of the attributes of a much more competitive market, and many new organizations were active in the market. However, something in the health care market still was amiss.

Primary Conclusion

There was ample evidence in the 1980s of an excess supply of physician specialists and acute care hospital beds. Nevertheless, the new health care financing organizations weren't able to contain costs consistent with these supply conditions. The rate of health care inflation, after appearing to slow momentarily in the '80s, continued to climb one and one-half times higher than general price increases. Health care providers' income also continued to grow in real terms. The rate of increase in health care costs was expanding, not diminishing as would be expected in a period of greater competition.

One could conclude, as I had earlier, that the private health care market had performed reasonably well up to 1965. My renewal of the project began by reexamining that conclusion. I reviewed the information to identify what went wrong in the health care marketplace prior to 1965 that might have caused excessive inflation in the Medicare period. After assuming that something had gone grossly wrong in the development of the market it was not difficult to identify the anticompetitive problems that are outlined in the book.

Anticompetitive behavior of doctors and hospitals, aided and abetted by insurance carriers and the federal government, was responsible for the dysfunctional growth of health care. The excess investment in high tech and specialized care was financed by "free" employer-sponsored, first-dollar health insurance coverage that consumers embraced without understanding the consequences. All of the post-1940 expansion in health care has been financed through growth in public and private health insurance. Consumers have become oblivious to the cost consequences of their health care purchasing decisions because the payment for these insurance programs—either taxes for the public programs or wages forgone for the private insurance—was almost totally separated from health care consumption decisions.

The Cost of Health Care Reform

Reform of the health care system cannot be accomplished unless consumers who are financially able are made accountable for their health care purchasing decisions. Neither market reform nor government regulation can be successful without the consumer's understanding of the benefits that will be derived from cost containment. Effective markets or effective market regulation both depend on the tensions that cost conscious consumer behavior brings to bear on competing health care suppliers. To control health care costs in the United States it is necessary to restore the consumer's role in health care decision-making. Consumers will neither seek lower-cost forms of health care or evaluate the efficacy of care in a free market nor permit regulators in a controlled market to discipline high-cost producers unless consumers are directly disadvantaged by inefficient producers charging excessive prices or providing unnecessary services. The study concludes with a reform proposal that could lead to sufficient consumer involvement in the health care market to control health care prices and restore a proper balance between health care consumers and providers. However, because the consumer's health care costs are currently concealed in employer-sponsored first-dollar, comprehensive health insurance benefits, any exposure of these costs will appear to be a loss of benefits to consumers when in fact it is simply a recognition of existing costs. Making this key point—consumers are currently bearing substantial excess but indirect costs for health care services—understood by consumers (voters) is the political dilemma that must be resolved in order to enact effective health care reform. Consumers can no longer afford more "free" health care.

History of Health Care

This is the principal lesson that has been learned by focusing on the economic implications of work done by historians of health care. Their work served as the basis for my interpretations of what has gone wrong in the economic development of the health care industry. Consequently, I owe a special debt to the substantial contributions of these predecessors, especially to Rosemary Stevens for her two fine books on the medical profession [1971] and on hospitals [1989]; to Anne and Herman Somers for their [1961] classic on doctors, patients, and health insurance; to Jon Kingsdale [1981] for his unpublished study of Baltimore hospitals; and to John Freymann [1974] for his tour de force on the health care system and scientific medicine. Their much more comprehensive analyses permitted me to concentrate on trying to understand why the health care market developed in such an eccentric manner without having to do my own original historical work. If my interpretation of the health care market has merit, the credit should go to the essential work of these predecessors. Any misunderstandings of their studies and consequent misinterpretations of the health care marketplace are solely my responsibility.

One significant benefit to readers of reviewing these and the other sources is to obtain a more balanced view of the participants in the development of the U.S. health care system. By focusing solely on the business of health care, I have necessarily slighted the importance of the roles of humanitarianism and social welfarism in health care. That part of the story is not told in this study, but it must be understood to judge the field's overall contributions to the quality of American life. All health care providers, whether individuals or organizations, function to help humanity, for which we should be thankful even though it sometimes has served as a rationale for avoiding the discomfort of market competition.

Dedication

This book is dedicated to two men who have served as my principal mentors in learning about the health care and public policy fields. Both served with great distinction as chief executive officers of the American Hospital Association. Edwin L. Crosby, M.D., Cy as he always identified himself in signing memos and letters, was a physician, public health officer, epidemiologist, and medical administrator. He served as administrator of Johns Hopkins Hospital, was the founding director of the Joint Commission on Accreditation of Hospitals (now the Joint Commission on Accreditation of Healthcare Organizations), and during his 18 years at AHA built the organization's capabilities both for helping hospitals better serve their communities and for honestly representing them to government and the public. J. Alexander McMahon, Alex, succeeded Dr. Crosby at AHA and for 14 years maintained the best of the Crosby traditions while vigorously and ably serving as the national advocate for hospitals during the difficult 1970s and early '80s. By education and inclination, Alex is a lawyer and teacher who also served during the early Medicare years as the CEO of the North Carlina Blue Cross and Blue Shield plan as well as chairman of the board of trustees of his alma mater, Duke University. My interest in health care and hospitals was initially sparked by Ed Crosby and then sustained and nurtured by Alex McMahon. They were successful in most respects, except for the transference of their patience and understanding of the timing of public policy actions, in teaching me how public health policy was formulated in this country. For both men's wisdom and perspective I owe a great deal.

Acknowledgements

Alex had the added burden of helping me with this study despite not fully concurring with its conclusions. Nevertheless, he is the only nonfamily member who has voluntarily read virtually all drafts of the manuscript. Perhaps that is why he suggested that instead of a full-fledged history the purposes of the book could be better served as a historical interpretation, which shortened it considerably and, even more important, permitted me to complete it. He, Stewart Hamilton, David Hitt, Jon Kingsdale, Bob Massey, Austin Ross, Rosemary Stevens, and Irv Wolkstein have helped with my original pre-Medicare history of hospitals. Alex, John Freymann, Don Dunn, and Andrew Drake helped sharpen my interpretation and arguments in the more recent work. Paul Pearson has painstakingly tried to straighten my fractured syntax by performing numerous copy edits of the various drafts. Eloise Foster and the AHA Resource Center staff have quickly and cheerfully responded to all of my reference requests. Winston Drake made it possible for me to master the use of a word processor and kept it going without the dreaded crash. John Samples, director of Georgetown University Press, did a remarkable job of getting the manuscript reviewed and published in record time. To all of those named and to other friends, I am most grateful for their help and encouragement.

Finally, my appreciation to my wife, Joyce, is immense for granting me the opportunity and support in all of my work demands. On this project I spent the work week on this idyllic dune overlooking Lake Michigan to ponder and pace while she labored in Chicago. In addition, thanks are deserved for her recognition of the personal importance to me of the project and constant encouragement that I might finally get it done.

*   *   *

Understanding the economic development and operation of the health care industry is not an easy puzzle to solve. Although I am sure some of the pieces are still not properly in place, I finish this project with the hope that a more orderly understanding of the industry has emerged. My concluding wish is that it will be sufficiently helpful in designing the needed reform of our nation's health care system.

April 1994   D.F.D.
Beverly Shores, Indiana.

1
History, Reform, and the Health Care Market

During the 1992 presidential campaign and in the first months of Bill Clinton's presidency, health care reform became one of the top priority issues for the United States. In various guises proposed federal legislation for financing health care services has been on the nation's congressional agenda since 1915. Over the nearly 80 years of consideration, the nature of these legislative proposals has differed, reflecting both changes in the character of national political activity and the state of the health care industry. However, never before has the passage of a federal financing system for health care seemed more likely, nor have the problems of providing and financing health care services been more complex.

The principal purposes of this book are (1) to review the economic history of health care in the United States during the 20th century in order to understand the nature and cause of the existing deficiencies in the health care marketplace, (2) to assess the adequacy of the proposed Clinton plan for health care reform, and (3) to propose additional reforms for remedying the market deficiencies.

In this chapter, the context and objectives of the current debate over health care reform is first described by comparing the 1990s debate with past reform efforts. The current reform effort is principally focused on repairing the defects in the health care market. An overview of the health care market is presented to identify the primary symptoms of failure in the health care market and the issues or market characteristics that need to be fixed. The objective of the study is to understand the historical reasons for these symptoms and be able to

1

evaluate the adequacy of the Clinton and other reform proposals to overcome the problems identified. Finally, a brief outline of the entire study is provided.

HEALTH CARE REFORM PROPOSALS

Past Reform Efforts

Although the general issue of public health insurance has, at least nominally, been on the nation's legislative agenda since 1915, Paul Starr [1982a], a Pulitzer prize-winning medical sociologist, has concluded that there were three separate phases of consideration for an expanded federal role in health with different objectives for each. In the first phase, at the conclusion of the progressive era, advocates of national (federal) health insurance sought "a program of income maintenance for wage earners and disease prevention" to increase national efficiency. This reform movement was an aberration in that it was more closely linked to the social insurance movement than to subsequent health care reform efforts that focused more narrowly on health care. The U.S. health care industry was in its infancy; major medical interventions were extremely risky; and wages lost during the patient's illness, not the cost of health care, was the primary concern.

The second phase, beginning prior to World War II and extending into the 1960s, sought to have the federal government develop a mechanism for "medical care financing to distribute individual risks and expand access" to care for lower-income groups. Health care costs were now significant, but the primary issue was making health insurance available to all citizens, not just the employed. The passage of a health insurance program in 1965 for the poor and the elderly, who were the most vocal and organized advocates of national health insurance (NHI), relieved the immediate political pressures for passage of a universal health insurance program.

Starr's third phase, which occurred in the 1970s after the implementation of the Medicare and Medicaid programs, added "a program of cost control and institutional reform as well as [the] universal coverage" objective envisioned in the previous phase. The rate of increase in health care costs had reached a new plateau as a result of the new federal programs for the poor and, especially, the aged. Many believed that only the federal government could provide sufficient leverage to control those burgeoning costs. However, government at all levels proceeded during the remainder of the 1970s, without NHI legislation, but with nearly three years of national wage and price controls over the health care industry, to exercise all of the traditional methods of governmental cost control with only limited success.

Health Care Reform in the 1990s

The Clinton plan for health care reform reflects and extends the objectives of all these past reform efforts. However, the size of the federal budget deficit has made consideration of health care as a part of a national social insurance program virtually impossible. Nevertheless, the public's general dissatisfaction with high health care costs and the rising middle class concern about continued employment and the consequent availability of health insurance have been the driving political forces for placing NHI so high on the legislative agenda. Since the Reagan revolution for limiting government and strengthening market discipline, the public rhetoric of the health care reform debate has changed. It is no longer being considered in terms of the traditional language of social insurance or even the 1970s language of a citizen's right to a cost-effective NHI program. Reform itself, rather than NHI, has become the central metaphor of the 1990s public debate. Reform, which in the past has been used to describe the entire historic movement for changing the health care delivery and financing system, now implies improving the existing system by alteration or removal of defects rather than building a whole new system.

The current popularity of the health care reform issue suggests a general agreement that the health care marketplace is broken and that restructuring that marketplace is necessary to fix it. Except for the social insurance advocates, there seems to be no mandate for a whole new government insurance program. However, because of other national problems with job creation and the federal deficit, it may also imply a broadening of reform goals to not only improve our citizens' access to health services and contain or even reduce health care costs, but also to protect or, if possible, improve employment opportunities and reduce the drain of health care expenditures on the federal budget.

Health care has grown to consume an ever larger share of the federal budget and our nation's output. Therefore, the political and economic importance of the health care industry has assumed greater relevance in public policy making. It is no longer sufficient to consider NHI only in terms of how a specific proposal will affect access, cost, and quality of health care in the United States; the proposal must also be considered in terms of how it will affect the national budget deficit, employment opportunities, and even national competitiveness in world markets.

The health care industry in the United States recently began to take on economic and political significance far beyond the concerns of health care consumers, hospitals, doctors, or the drug companies. Just as the auto, energy, or computer industries served as lightning rods for changes in the nation's economic development, the health care industry now has that spotlight. By commanding one-seventh of the nation's resources, providing one-eleventh of all jobs, and having central importance to all labor-management negotiations by being the most prized and vigorously defended labor fringe benefit for seven-eighths of all employed persons, the health care industry has an importance beyond its services for health.

President Clinton's identification of the general issue of security for all our citizens as a goal for the nation has generated much support. Security encompasses not only health care, but financial and job security for middle class and affluent Americans. Government itself, at all levels, is straining under the weight of the bill for health care services of its direct beneficiaries. In 1992 one-sixth of the federal budget and one-seventh of state budgets were committed to expenditure for health care services or research and development. Because nearly three-fourths of state and federal health care expenditures are made for the Medicare and Medicaid entitlement programs, the critical issues of federal control of its budget deficit and state supported activities for education, income maintenance, and infrastucture investment cannot be resolved without finding a solution to the health care spending conundrum.

The extraordinarily high rate of increase in health care spending over the last four decades has taken its toll on Americans not only in terms of insecurity about health care costs and insurance coverage, but also in terms of other spending alternatives that have had to be forgone or investments that could not be afforded. The central lesson of economics is that no nation can spend so much on one segment of the economy without having fewer resources to devote to other uses.

Thus, the current debate over health care reform requires both a narrower focus on the imperfections of the health care marketplace and a broader focus on the implications of health care spending on the rest of the economy. What is needed in this debate is, first, an identification of what has gone wrong in the health care market and then an analysis of the alternative remedies for repairing those flaws in the broad context of how these solutions will affect the general health of the American economy.

THE CURRENT STATE OF THE HEALTH CARE MARKET

David E. Rosenbaum [1993], a reporter for the *New York Times*, recently described the U.S. health care system as "America's economic outlaw" that defies the fundamental laws of supply and demand; a market in which oversupply leads to price increases instead of price reductions and new technology lowers productivity and raises costs; and health as such a priceless commodity that "people place no limit on what they will pay" for health care services. Although Rosenbaum's description may be slightly overdrawn (rather than "outlaw," it may only be a market that can't shoot straight), it certainly captures the public's popular impression of the health care market being out of control and in need of reform.

The rationale for a market strategy of health care reform is based on the belief that the health care market can be made more efficient. An efficient market allocates resources according to the preferences of consumers so as to maximize the total consumer satisfaction from the consumption of that level of resources. Its efficiency results from self-reinforcing incentives, the so-called "invisible hand," created by buyers and sellers competing to satisfy consumer preferences.

The first incentive is for consumers, operating with limited resources, to be sensitive to the price of alternative goods and services in selecting a market basket for consumption. In an efficient market, product prices strongly influence consumer choice. Consequently, producers of goods or services have a significant incentive to price their products as low as possible by controlling their production costs. It needs to be emphasized that pricing is only one of the ways in which producers compete with one another. The design and marketing of products according to consumer preferences are also important determinants.

The efficiency of a given market is judged by how well it allocates resources in accordance with consumer preferences and minimizes the quantity of resources consumed in meeting those preferences. Few actual markets come close to performing with perfect efficiency. Nevertheless, markets generally represent a very effective means for a society to choose which goods and services ought to be produced and to encourage their efficient production.

Despite the general effectiveness of most markets in our economy there are some notable exceptions. Economists have described the circumstances surrounding such markets as market failure. Markets may fail for a variety of reasons. When the impediments to a market's successful operation are basic or structural, alternative mechanisms, such as regulation or even direct government operation, are often viewed as necessary. The choice of an alternative mechanism to replace a free market depends on the kind of flaws perceived in that market.

Market failure is the economist's diagnosis of the health care industry, and the high rates of increase in health care costs are simply viewed as symptoms of a structural flaw. The market reform proponents, however, believe that the market can be restored to health by eradicating the impediments to essential market incentives for appropriate consumer and producer behavior rather than by alternative mechanisms such as regulation or complete governmental operation.

In order to understand the reasons for the renewed interest in health care reform, it will be helpful to outline the current problems of the health care marketplace. From a political standpoint, the fundamental problems are high cost and uneven access to health care. However, more technical indications suggest that the more fundamental problem from an economics standpoint is market failure. After a brief summary of the cost and access problems, the technical, economic characteristics of the health care market will be reviewed, first, to find out if there are any inherent structural difficulties in the health care market that preclude the successful operation of a competitive market, and second, to identify the symptoms or technical indications of market failure in health care that can serve as questions to be answered in the study's historical analysis of the U.S. health care market.

High Cost and Uneven Distribution of Services

Access to health care service in the United States has for the past several years been measured in terms of health insurance coverage rather than the availability of doctors and hospitals. Americans are more concerned about having health insurance benefits to reduce the financial barriers to obtaining health care services than they are about the availability and utilization of the services themselves. In the first decades after World War II, the concern about access focused on the shortage or geographic maldistribution of doctors and hospitals, especially in rural and inner-city communities.

The current concern suggests that the increased supply of physicians and hospital beds that began in the 1960s, as well as changing utilization patterns, redefine the access to care problem. Nevertheless, the primary reason for the increased American emphasis on insurance coverage was the substantial increase in the cost of health care. For example, an average stay in an acute hospital in the 1950s required just over two weeks of work for the median-income American family. In 1990 despite a lower likelihood of being hospitalized and a half-day shorter length of stay, that same median-income family had to work more than seven weeks to pay for an admission to an acute care hospital. The ratio of seven to two weeks of work required to pay the increased cost of a hospital stay over this 40-year period indicates that real cost of hospital care in terms of the amount of work effort required for a hospital stay has increased 3.5 times.

Since 1965, the percentage increase in the relative quantity of resources that the U.S. economy has devoted to health care services, as measured by health care spending as a percentage of gross domestic product, has risen more rapidly than spending on any other group of goods or services. In 1965 the allocation of GDP for health care was 5.9 percent; by 1993 that allocation had risen to nearly 14 percent. Although spending more on a particular service may simply reflect a change in consumer preference about health care services over time, there is substantial evidence that the U.S. market for health care reflects the changing preferences of health care providers, not the choice of the American consumer.

More frequently today than in the past, stories describing the wonders of modern medicine also emphasize the exorbitant costs of these miraculous cures. Medically-induced bankruptcies (the leading cause of personal bankruptcy) have become almost as important a news story as stories about medicine's powerful new therapies. For example, Barlett and Steele [1992] in their book on what's wrong in American devote an entire chapter to a series of stories about the personal tragedies of persons losing their jobs and their health insurance coverage. It is not surprising that American concern about the rising cost of health care services has produced a mass phobia. Persons with insurance coverage through employment are unwilling to change jobs for fear of losing that coverage (often called "job lock"), and have a near-paranoia about losing their jobs. Cooper and Monheit [1993] have documented a reluctance on the part of employees to change jobs for fear of losing health insurance benefits. As President Clinton has discovered in promoting the Clintons' health care reform proposal, security is the fundamental concern of the American people. In the 1990s Americans no longer worry about the availability of health services, but they are obsessed about their ability to pay for needed services because of the magnitude of health care costs. These high costs have altered the American view of what access to health care means and, in terms of the '90s' definition of access, the higher costs have contributed to a perceived lessening of insurance coverage for both the employed and the beneficiaries of government programs.

Higher health care costs are responsible for greater demand for health insurance and for an increasing number of Americans being priced out of the insurance market or receiving less adequate coverage. The percentage of Americans having some form of health insurance coverage, public or private, rose steadily since the inception of such insurance in the 1930s but peaked at 87.2 percent in 1988. Since 1989 the number of persons without health insurance has been increasing faster than the number of new enrollees. The breadth of health insurance coverage in aggregate, as measured by the percentage of personal health expenditures paid through insurance coverage, however, has continued to increase despite the rising number of persons without insurance and (or perhaps, because of) increased cost sharing by employees.

The average percentage of personal health expenditures paid by public and private insurance programs has continued to grow. Consequently, the percentage that has been paid by consumers directly for health care services at the time of service has been falling, especially rapidly since 1966. Although insurance has been paying a larger share of the bill, the amount of consumer payments for health care has been rising significantly—8 percent per year over the 25-year period—because the rate of increase in health care costs, more than 11 percent, has been greater than the growth in health insurance coverage. Therefore, health care costs, not the diminution of health insurance coverage, are posing a growing access problem for most Americans. Even the relative dollar amount of consumer expenditures, measured as a percentage of disposable income, has remained fairly stable over this 25-year period. In 1965 consumer expenditures for out-of-pocket health expenses and health insurance premiums represented 4.8 percent of disposable personal income, and in 1990 the percentage was 4.7 percent.

However, the lack of health insurance is a problem for a growing number. Table 1.1 presents some of the personal characteristics of this group of uninsured Americans. Columns 2 and 3 suggest that most uninsured persons have full-time employment, a high school education or better, come from a family earning more than $15,000 a year, and are white. However, column 4 (the percentage of that category without insurance) indicates that the probability of not having health insurance is greater for individuals without full-time employment, with lower levels of educational achievement and family income, and for minority races. This situation is especially unfortunate because the unemployed, the less well educated, the poor, and the racial minorities are more likely to have health problems requiring more, not less, care. Furthermore, when uninsured persons do make their way into the health care system, they are likely to receive inferior care [Burstin, et al, 1992].

There are at least two problems with access to health care in 1990s America. For employed, middle-class Americans, the access problem is the fear of job loss coupled with an illness that will require a high-cost medical technology for a family member that will result in a medical bankruptcy. Higher-income persons in 1990s America seem to view this access problem as having the potential for medical bankruptcy. There is no evidence that employed persons are, on average, making any significantly greater out-of-pocket health care expenditures relative to their disposable income. In other words, U.S. business conditions with high job uncertainty plus an awareness of the high cost of medical care has caused higher income Americans to question the acceptability of the current health care financing and delivery system. Support for an NHI program, financed totally by

TABLE 1.1　Status of Persons Without Health Insurance in 1990

Employment Characteristic	Number of Persons (millions)	Percent of Uninsured	Percent of Category
Full-time	19.3	54.3%	12.5%
Part-time	2.8	7.7	27.7
Mostly F-T	5.7	15.8	31.1
Part-year	2.8	8.0	26.9
Unemployed	5.2	14.5	22.6
Total	*35.8*	*100.0%*	
Education			
No high school	5.7	15.9%	37.7%
Some high school	6.0	16.8	27.1
High school grad	14.0	39.3	17.7
Some college	5.9	16.5	12.9
College graduate	2.5	7.1	8.5
Postgraduate	*1.6*	*4.5*	6.7
Total	*35.7*	*100.1%*	
Family income			
Under $5,000	4.5	12.7%	35.6%
$5,000–9,900	5.0	14.0	32.9
$10,000–14,999	5.7	15.9	35.5
$15,000–19,999	4.5	12.7	28.6
$20,000–29,999	6.5	18.3	19.3
$30,000–39,999	3.8	10.5	11.7
$40,000–49,999	2.0	5.7	7.8
$50,000 or more	*3.7*	*10.3*	5.7
Total	*35.7*	*100.1%*	
Race			
White	21.0	58.6%	13.1%
Black	6.2	17.4	22.8
Hispanic	7.0	19.6	34.8
Other	*1.6*	*4.3*	19.5
Total	*35.8*	*99.9%*	

Source: Kosterlitz [1992a, 385] based data from the Employee Benefit Research Institute.

government funds, has reached the highest level in public opinion polls of any time since World War II [Blendon and Donelan, 1990]. Obviously this middle-class access problem is significant for the molding of public opinion in the debate over health care reform.

The second access problem involves the uninsured poor who do not qualify for government assistance through Medicaid. If the American experience after the implementation of the Medicare and Medicaid programs in 1966 is indicative, increased investment in resources for health care of these persons could significantly improve their health. However, Medicaid eligibility for the poor has gotten worse in recent years. The problem of inadequate health insurance coverage for lower-income Americans has been with us for a long time, certainly since 1966, and therefore has probably not had a substantial effect on the recent change in general public opinion. However, health reform in the 1990s should address this access problem by including provisions for additional resources for under-employed, lower-income, less well-educated, and minority Americans.

Finally, it must also be recognized that increasing access to care for these more than 35 million Americans will exacerbate the already difficult health care cost problem for all Americans. The primary political problem with the American health care system is that health care costs are excessive as measured by the willingness of even affluent Americans to bear these costs. The fundamental political American health care problem is cost, cost, and cost.

Health Care Market Anomalies

In contrast to the magnitude of the political problem, there does not appear to be any overwhelming structural impediment in the health care marketplace to cause such frustration. Only two market anomalies have been identified that make the health care market differ substantially from economists' usual working assumptions about competitive markets. The primary anomaly is the substantial departure from the economist's assumption that the consumers have perfect knowledge of the benefits to be derived from the consumption of services. In practice, consumers have great uncertainty about the benefits that will be derived from the purchase of health care services. Without knowing what to expect from health services, both before and after consuming those services, the consumer could have difficulty in assessing (before) or evaluating (after) the appropriate price that should be paid and the quantity of services that should be purchased.

Imperfect knowledge of the health care benefits can be especially serious in dealing with the treatment of life-threatening injuries or illness when great emotional stress may surround the choice of treatment. However, the purchase of the vast majority of health care services does not involve such critical situations. Usually, the consumer looks to the physician to serve as an agent in the purchase of most health care services whether the need is critical or not. The dual role of advisor as to what the consumer should purchase and the provider of health care puts the physician in a unique position in the health care marketplace.

Trust between patient and physician may become a central part of the healing process and make characteristics of the market transaction of only secondary importance to the patient. Physicians are expected, and indeed pledge, to place the patient's well-being over their own economic interests. In many countries a dichotomy has developed between primary care physicians, who more actively serve as patient advisor while providing only basic diagnostic and therapeutic services, and specialty care physicians, who are available for referral by the primary care physicians to perform the more difficult and specialized diagnostic and therapeutic services. This dichotomy between primary and specialist care has not become the predominant organizational relationship in the U.S. health care market. In fact, one of the peculiarities of the U.S. health care market is the frequency with which patients directly select specialists or even request services from tertiary care institutions without physician referral.

Another issue that must be considered in evaluating competitive market solutions to health care reform is the effect "the dynamic tension [that is] found in most competitive markets" may have on "the production of good medical care" [Fuchs, 1969]. Concern about the degree and kind of competition that could evolve has prompted Arnold Relman, the editor emeritus of the *New England Journal of Medicine*, to crusade against the dangers of commercialism in medicine. It represents a valid concern as evidenced by the practice in the 1980s of some physicians who increased patient referrals to facilities in which they had invested. Such behavior could seriously damage the trust relationship between patient and physician, as well as unnecessarily increase health care costs.

Because of consumer uncertainty and the benefit of combining the advisory and provider roles, the physician had ample leverage to become the strong captain of the health care team—prescribing services and medications, admitting patients to the hospital or nursing home, and performing surgery or recommending surgery and surgeons. As a consequence, the practicing physician has virtually unchallenged control over the utilization of health care services. Therefore, the organization and the method of paying for the physician services are critical to the evaluation of reform proposals.

The physician's relationship of trust to the patient also implies that the economist's assumption of profit maximization may have limited relevance to the physician's patient decisions. In addition, the not-for-profit private and public institutions, which have made up the vast majority of the organizations providing institutional health care in the United States, further complicate the value of the profit motive as a means of predicting economic behavior in the health care market.

Hospitals, which are the largest and most expensive component of the modern health care delivery system, originally sprang from the charity motives of social welfare organizations. As the effectiveness of medical treatment grew, its emphasis changed to health care with social agency responsibilities. In many respects this change complemented the hospital's charity origins because the provision of care to the sick and injured was even more socially desirable as cures became more frequent. The success of modern medicine then brought the hospital into the marketplace because health care services became saleable to middle-class and more affluent buyers. Early in the 20th century revenues from patients, rather than philanthropic donations from patrons or organizations, became the principal financing source for the expansion of hospital services. Higher-income patients provided the resources for financing charity care. Cost shifting among different groups of patients is a long-established practice in hospital pricing.

Thus the hospital was shaped by three of its separate but linked missions. The first was humanitarian service and comfort to less fortunate members of society. Second, the provision of health care services eventually surpassed the hospital's original charity or community services because of the increased efficacy of medical science. Finally early in this century, the hospital became a marketplace business when the successes of modern medicine made Americans not only willing to enter what once were 19th century pesthouses but even willing to pay for the privilege.

Ironically, the hospital's three linked missions—charitable service, scientific medicine, and business enterprise—were never fully consistent and often represented competing goals. Shifting environmental pressures changed the balance of the three missions as the hospital developed in the 20th century. For instance, the managerial/ business role did not achieve prominence over its social agency mission until the 1930s. The Great Depression put such a high premium on financial acumen and successful management skills that trustees finally surrendered control of the hospital's day-to-day operations to professional hospital administrators. However, the business or economic mission in the not-for-profit private or governmental hospitals has rarely ever achieved parity with the predominant medical science mission.

In conclusion, the health care market's idiosyncrasies stem primarily from two sources: (1) the unevenness of knowledge between the physician/provider and the consumer, and (2) the restrictions on profit maximization behavior of physicians imposed by professional or agency considerations and on not-for-profit health care entities as a result of multiple and conflicting organizational missions. Despite the competing objectives and qualifications of the profit motive, economists, and with some success, have developed alternative models to explain or predict the economic behavior of these not-for-profit economic entities and have also constructed decision models for dealing with imperfect knowledge [Pauly, 1980]. Imperfect consumer knowledge and constraints on the profit motive also exist in varying degrees in other industries for which the competitive model has, nevertheless, proven analytically useful. The two anomalies in the health care market may have influenced market behavior and, hence, the development of the health care market in the United States, but certainly not to the extent of making the health care market an "economic outlaw" or even affecting the market's ability to shoot straight.

Current Symptoms of Market Failure

A number of symptoms of market failure have already been identified in our review of the health care market. First and most obvious, the costs of health are so high that general political agreement has been reached about the need for the federal government to reform the market. After decades on the congressional agenda, obtaining political consensus about the need for reform is a remarkable achievement and indicates the seriousness of the problem as a key symptom of market failure.

No other nation in the world has such high costs or spends as much of its GDP on health care as the United States. In chapter 6 a thorough comparison of U.S. costs with the health care costs of other developed nations reveals that one of the most important ways in which the U.S. health care system differs from other systems is its use of technology. The U.S. health care system is the most high-tech and specialized delivery system in the world.

Medical care in the United States is not organized into primary and specialist care to the extent that other nations have organized their health care delivery systems. The United States has fewer by far (less than one-third of all practicing physcans) primary care physicians and more specialists than other nations, which typically have a 50:50 ratio between primary and specialty care physicians. The relative lack of primary care physicians has market implications for carrying out the dual role of the physician in advising consumers while providing health care services. This finding may also suggest that in the U.S. health care market physicians have substituted their own preferences for the choices consumers would make if they had as much medical knowledge as the physicians.

Some U.S. health care consumers directly select their own specialists and even tertiary care hospitals without referral from either primary or specialty care physicians. This practice not only suggests that advisory/ counselling function role in purchasing health care is not working fully, it may also indicate that the health care consumer is freelancing without regard to the cost of care as a method of coping with the lack of physician counselling assistance in an orderly market for health care.

Developmental Symptoms of Market Failure

In addition to these three symptoms of market failure, two process symptoms can only be discovered by observing the health care market over time. The first process symptom is the slowness of the pace and unusual direction of market development itself. The second process symptom is the technical failure of the health insurance market.

Lack of Organizational Development

Most industry markets follow a fairly predictable pattern of development in four stages—introduction, growth, maturity, and decline—and each of these stages have had certain common characteristics [Porter, 1980]. During the introductory stage, the industry's product is of questionable quality, appeals only to a segment of the total potential market, and is often more expensive to produce because of the inability to substitute lower-skilled labor and to take advantage of operating at high levels of capacity. The growth phase differs from the introductory stage only in the accelerated rate of growth that occurs as a consequence of the product's broader acceptability in the marketplace through greater quality control, and hence higher quality/reliability, and lower production costs by substituting lower-cost labor and operating at more optimal levels of capacity. Maturity is attained for a product when the market has been fully saturated, technical quality is high but lower-cost substitute products of equal or higher quality become available, and industry capacity generally becomes excessive. An industry's decline occurs when more and even better substitutes become available, producing substantially larger excesses in the industry's capacity.

Health care in the United States experienced a fairly consistent and defined introductory phase. From the turn of the century to 1940 the development of quality and production standards and a method of marketing and financing of health care services were the major market organizing efforts. During and after World War II health care began a growth phase that continues today, although segments of the industry, such as hospitals, have reached the mature phase. Overall, the health care industry continues to grow at extremely high rates, and that is the problem that reform needs to address.

Health care has not passed through the succeeding phases of industry development, nor have the changing methods of producing health care over the 20th century realized any significant economies of scale or resulted in lower-cost production inputs, both of which might have reduced the cost of providing health care services. In fact, until quite recently there were no sizeable organizational or structural changes in the makeup of the industry that either improved product quality or reduced product costs. Since 1941 growth within a stable organizational structure has been the industry's fundamental pattern. Only in the late 1970s did that pattern appear to change, but even then this change did not clearly bring greater efficiency to the production of health services. Rationalizing the production of health care services certainly should be one of the objectives of health care reform. Perhaps the lack of profit maximization, or, more accurately, the substitution of multiple, albeit more humanitarian, objectives for hospitals reduces the competitiveness in the health care market by dulling the incentives for producer efficiency that are normally expected to operate in competitive markets. If the hospital, as the primary business enterprise in the health care market, is not seeking to minimize its operating costs, there may be implications for the overall effectiveness of the market.

Technical Failure of Health Insurance

The fifth symptom of market failure can best be seen by reviewing the historical development of the health insurance product. In the 1930s, actuaries from commercial insurance carriers questioned whether health insurance could be written in terms of first-dollar service benefits for several reasons: (1) there was no objective basis for estimating the insurable losses, i.e., little was known about the frequency or cost of various kinds of illness or injury; (2) the insured had better information than the carrier to assess the insurance risk, i.e., there was risk to the carrier of adverse risk selection in that those individuals who were more likely to experience higher health care costs were also more likely to purchase health insurance and vice versa; and (3) the presence of first-dollar health insurance could encourage greater health care utilization and higher costs. Consequently when commercial carriers entered the health insurance market, they wrote policies in terms of dollars of benefit per unit of service, imposed deductibles and coinsurance, and experience rated the groups purchasing the insurance as techniques for overcoming the three actuarial difficulties [MacIntyre 1962].

Today's huge health insurance industry no longer lacks sufficient data on frequency and cost to overcome the technical estimating problem. The evidence, however, supports the validity of the early actuarial concerns about the potential for adverse risk selection as well as health insurance inducing higher utilization. The Rand study, a multimillion dollar research project conducted over seven years ending in 1982, confirmed the higher utilization effect of insurance. It found that health care costs were nearly one-third less for persons with relatively large deductibles, or at least 25 percent coinsurance provisions, than those individuals having free care (first-dollar coverage). Furthermore, there was no observable effect on health except for lower-income families [Brooks et al 1983]. Although this finding in the United States is equally applicable to other developed nations that have governmentally-sponsored insurance programs with low or first-dollar coverage, its cost inducement implications are much more critical in a private market approach to controlling health care costs because the governmental insurance programs have other controls to regulate utilization, such as queuing as a result of limiting the supply of health care resources.

In addition, the actuaries' concern about risk selection has been borne out in findings that illnesses and accidents are not randomly distributed across the population. For example, Roos, Shapiro, and Tate [1989] found in a 16-year study that about half of the population will have few, other than routine, health care needs over their lifetimes, that another 45 percent will incur substantial lifetime health care costs, and that the remaining 5 percent will have extraordinary health care problems and expenses over their lives. This distribution of health care expenditures was found across all age groups and was consistent over time, which suggests that individual enrollees should have signficantly better information about their own health risks than do the insurance carriers.

With this underlying pattern for individual lifetime expenditures it is not surprising that the distribution of health care expenditures in any given year is even more concentrated. Berk and Monheit [1992] assembled the health expenditure data in Table 1-2 from several historical sources. These authors credit Aaron with the observation that "the concentration of health care expenditures creates 'enormous incentives' for private insurers to identify high-cost users of care and to keep their numbers to a minimum to ensure profitability and to

TABLE 1.2   Distribution of Health Expenditures for the U.S. Population By Magnitude of Expenditures for Selected Years between 1928–1987

% of U.S. Pop. Ranked by Exp.	1928	1963	1970	1977	1980	1987
Top 1%	—	17%	26%	27%	29%	30%
Top 5%	52%	41%	50%	55%	55%	58%
Top 30%	93%	—	88%	90%	90%	91%
Bottom 50%	—	5%	4%	3%	4%	3%

Source: Berk and Monheit [1992].

control premium costs." All insurers would like to insure the healthy half of the population and, even more important, avoid the unhealthy 5 percent, who account for more than half of health care expenditures in any given year, but only about one-quarter of the expenditures for their age cohorts over their lifetimes [Roos, Shapiro, and Tate, 1989].

The most obvious insurance practice for avoiding the liability for the high-risk individual was to experience rate and shift the risks back to the group being insured. The exclusion of preexisting conditions was originally employed to avoid the risk of individuals insuring only when they knew health care services would be needed. That tactic has come to be used to avoid insuring persons who are likely to be members of the unhealthy 5 percent. Many more subtle techniques are employed by insurers and HMOs to avoid enrolling individuals who are likely to be higher risk; e.g., choice of advertising vehicles, design of benefit structure, and location of clinic sites [Luft and Miller 1988]. Unfortunately, such techniques are also frequently practiced by employers in an effort to mimimize their group health insurance costs. The insurance carrier's methods of structuring health insurance to take advantage of this small segment of the population with the illness concentration seems to have more than compensated for the traditional disadvantage that the 1930s actuaries feared would make health care uninsurable. No doubt the basic unfairness of seeking to avoid insuring the people who most need health insurance has contributed to low public esteem for private health insurance companies.

Risk avoidance by health insurance carriers and employers is one of the most serious social disruptions built into the current health care market. Their tactics for avoiding the high-risk individual are largely responsible for employee job lock and increased insecurity about continued employment. In addition, the concentration of high health care costs among few individuals is the cause of higher health insurance premiums for smaller groups. The probability for enrolling high-risk persons into an insurance group is virtually the same regardless of size, but only in larger groups can the increased costs of the high-risk individuals be spread across a sufficiently large number of enrollees that the premium cost will approach the average cost of health care in the community. Small groups and individuals are likely to have higher average health care costs and, consequently, are charged higher premiums than larger insurance groups. The higher premium cost results in fewer small businesses insuring their employees, which is the primary reason that more than half of all uninsured Americans are employed. In addition, first-dollar health insurance coverage certainly has contributed significantly to the high rate of health care cost inflation by lessening consumer incentives to be cost conscious in their purchase of health care. The design of health insurance is greatly in need of reform.

THE STUDY

The objective of this study is to understand why health care costs in the United States are so high and which of the four symptoms—physician over-specialization and overprescription of high-tech care, lack of consumer cost consciousness, ineffective industrial organization and stunted economic development, and flawed health insurance design—are genuine flaws that have contributed to market failure and excessive health care cost increases. The general thesis of the study is that one these four symptoms, flawed health insurance design, is the principal cause of failure in the health care market. Consequently, understanding how these symptoms arose in the development of the market and why the structure of health insurance represents a serious defect in the operation of the health care market will be helpful to evaluating reform proposals.

The next four chapters describe the economic development of the American health care industry. By contrasting that development with the pattern of development that has typified other American industries, the study amplifies the conclusions summarized in this chapter and points out additional problems in the health care market.

Chapter 2 describes the entry into the marketplace of the first health care firm, the hospital; how the scientific school of medicine gained control of the medical profession's education standards and thus the future of medicine; the alliance that was made between scientific medicine and the large urban and teaching hospitals to exclude GPs and other primary care physicians from the workshop of scientific medicine; and the revolt by the GPs, led by the AMA, to limit health insurance in the United States to noncompetitive plans by insisting on freedom of choice of physician and, consequently, fee-for-service medicine. That introductory phase of development, which lasted from 1900 to 1940, may well have been shorter if the United States had not experienced such a severe economic depression beginning in 1929 and extending through the 1930s. The health care industry grew in real terms during the Great Depression and was on the verge of even more substantial growth just prior to World War II.

Chapter 3 describes the industry's the first growth phase in which private health insurance and hospitals played the pivotal roles in industry development and covers the period from 1941 to 1965. This period was one of great coalescing of doctors, hospitals, and insurers around the organizational structure that had been created in the earlier phase of development. Key to the solidarity and stability of the industry's organization was support from the federal government both with assistance in making health insurance a part of collective bargaining and direct grant support for health facilities, research, and education. However, the primary reason for the industry's economic and political successes was the popularity of scientific medicine with the nation's consumers; scientific medicine had developed into a uniquely successful product, as typified by the antibiotic or wonder drugs.

Chapter 4 describes how that popularity led in 1965 to the enactment of Public Law 89-97, which amended the Social Security Act to provide public health insurance for the poor and the elderly. The model for the legislation had been the employer-provided, freedom of physician choice, "first-dollar" health insurance coverage that had been imprinted on the consumer in the post-war period. When that model was applied, without any additional cost controls, to the aged, who had always been the age group most in need of health care, the industry entered a second and exaggerated growth phase that permitted such an unobstructed flow of resources into the industry that its capacity soon swelled to more than Americans could easily consume.

Chapter 5 describes the second stage of that second growth phase, which the industry is still experiencing and is the catalyst for the current reform efforts. During that stage the alliance between hospitals and their medical staffs finally ruptured, health insurers assumed a more aggressive, price discounting strategy, but consumers remained only passively involved in the health care market.

Chapter 6 compares the performance of the current U.S. health care system with those of other developed nations to demonstrate and quantify the nation's overinvestment in medical science and technology. The history of the industry's development is then reviewed to identify the reasons for the failure of the U.S. health care market and to serve as a basis for evaluating the Clinton and other health care reform proposals.

Chapter 7 compares the Clinton proposed solutions with how a more effective market would have worked and presents some recommendations for strengthening the Clinton plan for health care reform. It concludes by presenting a quite different alternative for reforming the health care market that would fix the flaws that have been identified in this historical study of the U.S. health care marketplace, but may be less politically popular than proposals currently under consideration in Congress.

2
Establishing a Market for Health Care Services, 1900–1940

This chapter describes how centuries-old charitable hospitals combined forces with physicians to become the first successful health care business enterprise. The cumulative advances in scientific knowledge and understanding of the human body produced a new discipline—scientific medicine—and the need for a new, stronger institution in which that new discipline could practice—the hospital. Reaching an accord between physicians trained in scientific medicine and the old charitable hospital was an essential first step in the production of safer and higher quality institutional health care services that would appeal to the broad market of potential consumers of inpatient care.

When doctors and hospitals had attained reasonable success in producing marketable health care services, they needed an effective way to market and finance their services. This need sparked the initial efforts in the 1930s to establish an insurance program for hospital and physician services. A new type of accord between hospitals and doctors was required to fashion the health insurance product to their mutual satisfaction.

CREATING THE INSTITUTIONAL HEALTH CARE MARKET
1900–1929

The only market for health care services until the latter part of the 19th century had been for the personal services of physicians, dentists, and nurses. Because of its primitive nature at this time, the practice of medicine or dentistry was not very lucrative or prestigious. Consumers decided when to obtain these personal services, who would provide those services, and how much they were willing and able to pay. Charitable health care services were available to the poor, often through hospitals and charity clinics. However, most health care services were controlled by market forces, not by nonmarket administrative arrangements. Furthermore, these services were provided by a cottage industry similar to that for textiles prior to the industrial revolution. Perhaps the only real difference was that doctors and nurses provided many of their services directly in the consumer's home. Hospitals, on the other hand, were not yet subject to market control but were part of administrative arrangements made by local governments or private community or religious organizations to dispense charity services.

A modern marketing manager probably would have been unwilling to accept the assignment in 1900 of trying to sell hospital inpatient services to the vast middle-class market. The image of the 19th century hospital as a place for dying, a pesthouse inhabited by the dregs of society, was so unsavory that no modern Madison Avenue advertising campaign could have recruited middle-class patients, even for free care. The business payoff of the miracle of modern scientific medicine came about through the gradual reversal of the hospital's image from that of death and doom to one of hope and healing. By the late 1920s patients from all classes of society were utilizing the hospital and, as part of the American tradition of self-dependence, willingly paid for the cost of their care to the extent they were able. The commercial success of the hospital in the market economy only proved the old business adage that a good product will eventually sell itself.

The Product—Scientific Medicine

However, what consumers were willing to purchase was not hospital care, but care provided in hospitals by practitioners of the new discipline of scientific medicine. Although the cumulative effect of advances in scientific medicine in the second half of the 19th century significantly improved the hospital product, being an inpatient at the turn of the century was still far from a safe experience. A noted medical observer [Gregg 1956, 13] has recounted that it was not until 1910 or 1912 "when it became possible to say of the United States that a random patient with a random disease consulting a doctor chosen at random stood better than a fifty-fifty chance of benefiting from the encounter." Nevertheless, various well-trained physicians were practicing scientific medicine in the 1890s and early 1900s, and news began to spread about some miraculous cures accomplished in hospitals, which raised the hopes of the infirm. Actually, scientific medicine at the turn of the century provided few successful therapies beyond the provision of safer surgery, but "the mood of medicine was optimistic" [Stevens 1989, 18]. This rising perception of the benefits of modern medicine was as responsible as real product improvements in increasing the demand for scientific medicine practiced in the acute inpatient care hospital.

The hospital as a health care institution, not unlike other American business enterprises, emerged from a series of scientific discoveries—anesthesia in the 1840s, antisepsis in the 1860s, and x-ray and clinical laboratories in the 1890s. These and other discoveries required "bulky, expensive equipment which functioned only, or at best, in close proximity to the patient" [Kingsdale 1981, 81–82]. Thus doctors and patients were drawn to the hospital as the site for using the new technologies. The use of the x-ray, and later electrocardiography, was at first only practical in hospital facilities, and the need for antiseptic conditions moved surgery from the kitchen table to the surgical suite.

Although these technological innovations frequently were visualized as pieces of equipment or machines in hospitals, much more important to the provision of health care was the improvement in knowledge of the human body and the illnesses that invaded it. Major breakthroughs came from Pasteur's germ theory and Lister's application of antisepsis to surgery, both of which were applied directly to hospital care with tremendous improvements in the safety and productivity of patient care.

The growth in Europe, especially in Germany, of the applied sciences of bacteriology, physiology, anatomy, and pharmacology from the new discoveries in biology, chemistry, and physics was applied to the study of medicine. Curriculums for the study of scientific medicine unfolded quickly to revolutionize medical education in Europe. Despite the significant flowering of the American collegiate educational system after the Civil War, only a few great universities in the United States had anything resembling satisfactory opportunities for physician education. Many of the physicians who brought the newly discovered science to American medicine were themselves educated abroad. "Between 1870 and the outbreak of World War I, about 15,000 American physicians studied medicine in Germany alone" [Brown 1979b, 72]. Just as Francis Lowell had brought the factory system to America by pirating the power loom from the English, the study and practice of scientific medicine was imported from Europe.

The U.S. revolution in medical education sprang out of the experiment at Johns Hopkins, which had opened its doors to students in 1893. The study of medicine became a postgraduate program under the tutelage of four young physicians, two of whom had been trained in Germany and a third in Great Britain. The curriculum had a heavy emphasis on laboratory science in the first two years followed by clinical training in the hospital for the second two years. The American version of scientific medicine would extend more rigorously the precepts of objective clinical analysis, disease classification, and, especially, specialization of physician expertise for disease treatment than the European scientific practice models.

This more rigorous interpretation was not without its tradeoffs. For example, in the American interpretation the study of public health was excluded from the medical school curriculum and preventive care was neglected in the practice of the American version of scientific medicine [Freymann 1974, 46–47]. Instead it glorified objectified clinical analysis to classify patients into disease categories, which replaced the patient as the focus of analysis. As the noted clinician Dr. Stanley Joel Reiser [1993] has observed:

> Illness was now disease. The validity of particular symptoms depended on the capacity to state them as quantitative and pictorial indexes. Taken as a whole, developing a portrait of a medical problem was increasingly less the province of the patient, and more the prerogative of the physician.

However, the effect on medical practice of this increased emphasis on scientism and objectivity would not be observed until after World War II when the cumulative influence of other reinforcing factors, such as the model of health insurance that became primary, making this tendency even more pronounced.

Improving the Quality of the New Product

The first priority for the practitioners of scientific medicine, as it is with the developers of any new product, was to establish standards for improving their new medical product. The problem of product quality was enormous because the explosion in medical knowledge created such wide variations in the quality of physicians practicing medicine in the United States at the turn of the century. There were at that time nearly 134,000 physicians, or about 17.3 physicians per 10,000 population—a physician-population ratio that would not be reached again for more than 75 years. Unfortunately, only a small fraction of this large pool of physicians was qualified by rigorous education to practice scientific medicine.

It is difficult to estimate how many of the physicians practicing in 1900 had satisfactory medical training, either in the few good American schools or through study abroad. However, the number must have been quite small for Abraham Flexner's famous report[1] found few qualified physicians serving on medical school faculties at the time of his surveys. Unfortunately, most of the unqualified doctors had many years remaining in which to practice. Each year some of the incompetent retired and a larger number of graduates from the reformed medical schools increased slightly the percentage of competent physicians. However even by optimistic projection, it would be well into the 1930s before parity in the number of competent and incompetent physicians would be reached.

The medical profession was faced with an acute problem of technological obsolescence within its own ranks. The leadership of scientific medicine, who were aware of the gross deficiencies of most of their peers, felt an obligation to limit the practices of the inferior majority to avoid injuring the public without at the same time discrediting the entire profession. The option of starting over with the establishment of a new profession meeting the new standards of scientific medicine really was not attractive because the medical profession had been through a great public struggle in the last half of the 19th century over state medical licensure. The regular or allopathic physicians had tried to exclude homeopathic, eclectic, and other physician sects from licensure, but with only limited success. It was "only through the combined efforts of the regular and 'irregular' profession [that] laws could be secured to restrict medical practice to scientifically trained physicians" [Brown 1979a, 89]. Furthermore, the irregular medical therapies, principally herbal, were safer and often as effective until the recent advances in medical knowledge made their way into allopathic practice. Grandfathering became the means of accommodating the various medical sects and levels of competency.

The primary response to the medical competency problem was to cut off the flow of poorly trained new physicians by closing the inferior medical schools and by raising the medical education standards in the remaining schools. However, reforming the profession's education standard first required coalescing the profession in one strong organization, the American Medical Association, and then getting the AMA to lead the public battle for higher medical education standards. In the 19th century advocates for scientific medicine participated in many small elitist societies or associations [King 1983a and 1983b], and the AMA had only 8,400 members of the 134,000 physicians in the United States in 1900. After only a few years of active efforts, the reformers, gaining the support of the state medical associations, passed a major reorganization of AMA in 1901 and replaced its executive director with the editor of the association's journal, a physician sympathetic to the views of scientific medicine.

In 1903 the AMA put the dispute between regular and irregular physicians behind the profession by abandoning its previous position of excluding physicians trained as homeopaths or eclectics. In 1904 the Council on Medical Education was formed, and the reform of medical schools began in earnest. Initially, the new council conducted its own survey of the schools, but it subsequently arranged to have the Carnegie Foundation fund an "independent" survey by Abraham Flexner. By 1910 AMA membership had reached 70,000 members, and reform leadership maintained control until World War I. Brown [1979a] and Markowitz and Rosner [1979] describe these developments in the AMA. However, once the whole medical educational system had been redirected to a curriculum that was consistent with the precepts of scientific medicine the eventual success of the advocates of scientific medicine in controlling the profession was inevitable.

In 1910 Flexner's report was issued, and it made the Hopkins experiment the model for American medical education. His report presented a "merciless attack on contemporary medical education," especially "'commercial' medical schools—proprietary schools set up and run by physicians" [Brown 1979a, 133] without adequate admissions standards or lab facilities. The effect of the report was devastating to most medical schools. "Between 1904 and 1915, ninety-two schools merged or closed their doors in the face of higher state board requirements, financial difficulties, or adverse publicity . . . By 1915 the number of schools had been reduced to ninety-five . . . In 1905 only five schools had required any college preparation for admission. Ten years later eighty-five prescribed a minimum of one or two years' college preparation . . ." [Stevens 1971, 68]. The revolution in medical education begun at Hopkins drove "American medical science . . . from mediocrity to eminence, paving the way for world leadership in medicine in the years following World War I."

Stevens [1971] summarizes a number of other national organizational developments, including the establishment of the Association of American Medical Colleges and the formation of the National Board of Medical Examiners with increased support for a national examination for entrance to the profession. The aim of all these organizational changes was to raise state licensure requirements for the practice of medicine, which was gradually accomplished by state legislative actions. Inasmuch as all these efforts, except the establishment of the national board, preceded the publication of the Flexner report, the national leaders of the profession must have recognized the magnitude of the medical standards problem. King [1984, 1084] agrees that "the Flexner report was not in any sense an independent survey. It was initiated by the AMA with a specific goal in mind, to strengthen the hand of the Council [on Medical Education] in its dealings with the medical schools and the public."

Some economists and other historians have argued that these turn of the century efforts by the profession were motivated "to restrict supply in order to maintain and increase their price and profits" [Markowitz and Rosner 1979, 190]. Taken as a whole, however, the campaign by the advocates of scientific medicine immediately increased the number of licensed practicing physicians by including all of the physician sects. The reduced number of medical school graduates would affect the number of practicing physicians only gradually over many years. At that time there were very compelling reasons other than economic self-interest for raising the profession's entrance requirements. Those reasons stemmed from the explosion in medical knowledge and the consequential need for training that would equip the profession to practice scientific medicine. Of course, it is much easier to change behavior when that change is consistent with the underlying economic interests of the profession. However, action consistent with self-interest is a far cry from self-interest as the primary motive.

Relevance to Health Care Reform

Nevertheless, this episode, in which a small elite group of physicians reached an agreement with the vast majority of the medical profession by trading an inclusive licensing standard through grandfathering for control of the future medical education standards and, hence, important future product improvements, became the precursor of a consistent behavior pattern in the health care market at each stage of development. These leaders were willing to reduce their own lifetime incomes in order to strenghten the scientific basis of the profession's future practitioners. The alternative, i.e., to compete with the unqualified members of the profession by exposing their lack of competence, could have seriously delayed the public's understanding and acceptance of the new health care benefits of scientific medicine, as had been demonstrated by the public's confusion in the profession's struggle over licensing standards.

The consistent developmental pattern has been to choose the easiest, most accommodating, and least competitive option for structuring the health care marketplace. Eventually, all of the participants— physicians, hospital administrators, insurance executives, employers, employees, unions, and government officials—involved in the development of health care have acted in a manner consistent with their own self-interest, but tempered by a spirit of accommodation to the interests of others. Whether or not this accommodation was intended to reduce competition in the industry, it always seemed to have that effect. Only infrequently has such behavior maximized the self-interest of a single player to the detriment of others.

Unfortunately, such self-maximizing behavior has been increasing, probably as a result of the cumulative effect that these accommodations have had in lessening market discipline over the production and consumption of health care services in the United States. In other words, the spirit of accommodation that marked the development of the health care market is being replaced by greater emphasis on maximization of each group's self-interest. This observation suggests that, although reform is urgently needed, it has been and will continue to be increasingly difficult to accomplish.

Developing the Practice Site for Scientific Medicine

The second highest priority in the development of scientific medicine was the selection or construction of a site for practicing the new form of medicine. Because of the facility requirements for laboratories, x-rays, and antiseptic operating rooms, a hospital was needed; but what kind of hospital would be selected. The early practitioners of scientific medicine could have built and operated their own proprietary hospitals and captured the monopoly profits that have normally accrued to product innovators in other industries or they could have chosen to utilize the community resources, the not-for-profit hospitals, that had been created to care for the poor before the emergence of scientific medicine.

Although a survey conducted by the U.S. Bureau of Education in 1873 identified only 178 hospitals of all types in the entire country, Stevens [1989] estimated that there could have been as many as 4,000 hospitals in 1910. Of that number 1,500 to 2,000 were proprietary hospitals, i.e., for-profit hospitals owned by private parties, generally physicians or surgeons. These proprietary hospitals were typically very small institutions with a few beds for use by successful surgeons for wealthier patients who chose not to enter larger urban hospitals or for small-town doctors to practice in communities where capital was scarce, mainly in the southern and western parts of the United States. Most hospital care, despite the larger number of proprietaries, was provided in local governmental, religious, or private community institutions that were much larger and were better equipped. By 1904, these not-for-profit hospitals annually admitted more than one million patients with an average length of stay of 25 days and an average occupancy of 48 patients at the start of the year.

The climate was conducive to local efforts to expand hospital facilities, especially in growing urban areas. Also contributing to the expansion of hospital demand was the increasing difficulty faced by urban families in caring for their sick relatives. The extended family was no longer predominant, and urban housing was not suitable for caring for the ill. Per capita income rose after the economy recovered from the depression of 1893, and in general times were good following

America's triumph in the Spanish American War. Theodore Roosevelt was president during the beginning of a progressive era that extended to World War I. In addition, there were few constraints to establishing new hospitals in this period, except for rising capital costs, because there were few legal or professional standards for operating a hospital.

There were few market impediments to prevent practitioners of scientific medicine from choosing the profit-maximizing option to expand the number and size of the physician-owned hospitals as the principal site for their practice. Instead these physicians followed the evolving pattern of negotiating a less competitive agreement as an alternative to making for-profit hospitals the dominant hospital model in this new and growing industry. The not-for-profit hospital became the principal site for the practice of scientific medicine as a result of an accommodation reached with the trustees of the not-for-profit charity hospitals that for the first time permitted physicians to charge for services rendered in the charitable institution and granted an independent set of governing rules for the medical staff to control all medical affairs within the institution, subject only to the governing board's pro forma ratification. The effect of this arrangement was to make the hospital the physician's workshop, which restricted the amount of integration in health care services that would occur in most local markets. Although it was rarely challenged through antitrust litigation, it had many of the effects of the classic case of producers dividing markets to their mutual benefit, for most physicians until the 1970s and '80s did not organize competing health care services. The agreement also had a significant effect on the struggle by the technically competent practitioners to gain control of the site of major medical interventions into the human body.

In addition, it had profound effects on the growth of hospitals. Kingsdale's study [1981] of Baltimore hospitals, Vogel's [1980] of Boston, and Rosner's study [1979] of health care in Brooklyn all conclude that the growth of patient revenues during this period inexorably changed hospitals from predominantly charitable organizations to business organizations that looked to paying patients to help finance charity care. The metamorphosis of the charitable hospital into a business entity with a pressing need to expand market operations to continue charity services was remarkably swift. By the 1920s the new style was firmly fixed, and the competition for paying patients grew more intense among private hospitals. Philanthropic gifts were no longer used solely to finance the cost of charity care but also to purchase plant and equipment to modernize and expand patient services. As a consequence of this competition for paying patients, the physicians on the hospital's medical staff assumed the power and authority formerly held by the hospital's trustees. The physicians already had begun to change the balance of power within the institution as the growth in scientific medicine required physician autonomy in controlling the hospital's medical affairs. Furthermore, the 20th century method of financing hospital operations caused hospitals to become almost totally dependent on physicians. Trustees could still help to provide management expertise and tap philanthropic resources in the community, but those resources were now used to enhance the physician's workshop, not to expand charity care.

The hospital-medical staff agreement was not totally one-sided for hospitals profited from the scientific revolution in many ways. First, the improvements in the quality and safety of its product as well as the expansion in the kinds of surgical and medical interventions that were possible on an inpatient basis substantially increased the demand for medical staff appointments by physicians and the demand for inpatient care by consumers. Second, medical education, both undergraduate and graduate, introduced into many hospitals whole new product lines of medical education and research. Physicians in hospital training would become a new human resource in producing hospital services, just as student nurses had become a chief source of nursing services earlier. Third, these expanded activities produced a greater demand for capital facilities and equipment, which further centralized the practice of scientific medicine within the walls of the hospital and expanded the hospital's need to finance these capital acquisitions.

Specialization for Product Differentiation

Specialization, which was one way for the competent physician to become separated from the incompetent, became in the American brand of scientific medicine the rule rather than the exception. By 1929 there were more than 22,000 full-time specialists in a total of about 150,000 doctors. Since 1900 the whole profession had grown only by 16,000 doctors, and these newly educated physicians were overwhelmingly choosing specialization. This pattern of choice would continue. Although the expectation of greater economic rewards undoubtedly contributed to the choice of specialization, reducing the physician's level of uncertainty by focusing on a particular part of the human anatomy or a narrower set of procedures was also important.

While attempting to control the appointment of medical staff in individual hospitals, the "best" doctors also sought to develop national programs and strategies that could assist them in their local efforts. The establishment of specialty groups and credentialing individual physicians as specialists was helpful because such credentials provided a rational, defensible mechanism for administering hospital appointments and defining staff privileges. Furthermore, the specialist examinations could provide an incentive for physicians untrained in scientific medicine to renew their medical training and thus gain competency.

The founding of the American College of Surgeons in 1912 and, to a lesser degree, the American College of Physicians in 1915 were part of this response. The surgeons were especially concerned about the restriction of surgical privileges to competently trained surgeons, but they also accepted a major responsibility for upgrading the skills of their less well-trained colleagues. In 1918 the surgeons took on the assignment for the entire medical profession of developing a standardized accreditation program for hospitals, a program that in 1952 became the Joint Commission on Accreditation of Hospitals and subsequently changed its name to the Joint Commission on Accreditation of Healthcare Organizations, JCAHO.

The many specialty societies and the subsequent development of 20 medical specialty boards, beginning in 1917 with the ophthalmologists and to the 1969 founding of the family practice specialty, were related in varying degrees to a concern about medical competence. However, each specialty had its own political and economic concerns that often overshadowed the issue of competency. Despite an abysmal failure of some so-called specialists to qualify for practicing any branch of medicine in the armed services during World War I, the American Medical Association "had no means of controlling the numerical [or competency] balance between those content to be general practitioners and those striving toward specialization" [Stevens 1971, 131].

During the 1920s the AMA conceded much of its leadership over graduate medical education to the specialty boards, which in the early 1930s established coordination through their own Advisory Board for Medical Specialties rather than through the AMA's Council on Medical

Education. The AMA became the profession's political and economic spokesman and especially championed the cause of the general practitioner, who was by then "threatened by increased specialization . . . by the hospital as a potential center for medical elite . . . [and] by the public's growing interest in standards of medical care" [Stevens 1971, 147].

Physician Competition for Control of the Hospital

As the demand for health care increased, competition intensified between physicians who practiced mostly in and controlled hospitals and general practitioners who practiced a simpler style of medicine outside the hospital. This competition was marked by fee-splitting arrangements in which specialists, primarily surgeons, with hospital appointments would be asked to pay rebates to general practitioners in exchange for patient referrals. One of the first professional objectives of the newly established medical specialty groups, especially the American College of Surgeons, was to ban such "unethical" fee-splitting arrangements for their members.

The most crucial issue in the competition between advocates of scientific medicine and general practitioners was whether hospitals in same market area would have closed or open medical staffs. A closed staff was restricted to physicians admitted to membership by the hospital's organized medical staff. An open staff permitted membership of all practicing physicians in the community, but their practice privileges could be prescribed based on their credentials. Although the debate was waged in terms of protecting the public, the issue may have had greater significance for competition among physicians. The closed staff proponents argued that only qualified physicians should be given staff appointments. The open staff advocates claimed that medical standards in the community would be raised by allowing the hospital's medical staff to supervise the care provided by all physicians in the community.

In general, the outcome of the open versus closed staff dispute was largely determined by the market's population density.[2] Urban market areas had a preponderance of closed staff hospitals with most physicians having either no or single hospital admitting privileges. In nonurban areas where there were fewer specialists, the GPs fought for and frequently obtained open hospital staffing and, consequently, the right to admit patients to hospitals. Because the United States was becoming more urbanized, the specialists gained the most. The larger and most prestigious hospitals came under the control of closed staffs and, consequently, were controlled by advocates of scientific medicine and specialists. They also earned substantially more income than GPs.

The competition between physicians with hospital-based practices and those without hospital privileges in urban areas often reflected a basic difference in medical knowledge and competence. Physicians practicing in hospitals were presumed to be graduates of medical schools steeped in the tradition of scientific medicine. Although there is strong evidence that a great disparity in medical skills existed between the two classes of physicians, there is little evidence today that hospital staff appointments guaranteed that only scientifically elite doctors obtained hospital privileges and only those with inferior education were denied appointment in urban hospitals. Some of the for-profit hospitals organized during this period, especially in urban areas, were developed by physicians who did not have staff privileges in the not-for-profit hospitals. It is not clear to what degree these hospitals were established to correct inequities resulting from denial of privileges to scientifically trained physicians or to obtain practice privileges beyond the physician's skills. In the more rural and poorer areas, the for-profit, physician-owned hospitals were established because physician-invested funds were the only available source of capital.

In small or rural communities multiple staff appointments and open staffing became the predominant pattern. In general, cooperation rather than competition among physicians characterized the medical practice environment. Only rarely did the impassioned fire of professional jealousy that was very common in urban areas flare up in rural America. However, the quality of medical care was less scientifically sophisticated and undoubtedly of a lower standard than care rendered in urban practice.

During this period, the struggle within the house of medicine did not deter the emergence of the hospital as the site of scientific medicine. The relative desirability of a particular hospital's facilities was very important in the competition among hospitals in recruiting physicians. It also may have encouraged the medical elite to bring some procedures into the hospital that could have been accomplished more economically on an outpatient basis. Making these procedures part of the inpatient regimen, at least in urban areas, may have helped to protect them from abuse by the less competent. The hospital was becoming the sole community agency that provided some quality controls over the practice of medicine.

Hospital Economics and Finance

During the first three decades of the 20th century the hospital product line expanded, and the method of financing hospital services became more businesslike. Surgery under anesthesia and antiseptic conditions flourished. The safe opening of the abdomen and the pelvic area to surgery, with the death rate from these surgical procedures falling from 40 percent in the 1880s to less than 5 percent by 1900, was typical of the advances that made surgery the greatest growth product by far [Stevens 1989].

The increasing demand for hospital care, spurred by surgical advances, resulted in substantial hospital growth. Growth in hospital beds in the 19th century had stemmed primarily from increases in the size of the few existing institutions. Growth in the 1890s and the first part of the 20th century resulted from a significant increase in the number of institutions, thus causing the average size of hospitals to decrease [Kingsdale 1981, 180]. The total number of general hospitals grew to more than 4,500 at the end of the '20s with many smaller hospitals closing and more new ones opening.

Philanthropy alone could not have supported such a level of growth. The key to financing this expansion was the willingness of patients to pay for hospital care. Although white-collar workers and the upper class had always been expected to pay for necessary inpatient hospital services, the frequency of their utilization of hospitals increased markedly during this period. In addition, the advances in surgery prompted the working-class patients to begin to pay for hospital care. Hospitals responded to these new middle-class patients with new types of accommodations called "semi-private" to differentiate them from the charity patient wards and the private facilities of the well-to-do [Kingsdale 1981, 176–178].

"Data for hospitals around the country indicate that between 1889–90 and 1922 patient payments increased from less than one-third to two-thirds of operating expenses" [Kingsdale 1981, 239–240]. The growing importance of patient revenue was further magnified by substantial increases in hospital costs as the technological sophistication of the hospital product grew. Kingsdale [1981, 242] cites a more than 60 percent increase in per diem inpatient costs at Johns Hopkins between 1890 and 1920. Thus, paying patients were expected to cover not only the rising cost of their own hospital care, but many were also asked to contribute to the cost of charity care by paying charges that exceeded the cost of their own care.

By the late 1920s the hospital industry had became fairly large. In 1928 there were 6,852 registered hospitals in the United States with 892,934 beds and a capital investment of just over $3 billion [Rorem 1930, 25]. General hospitals made up about two-thirds of the total number of hospitals and had over 40 percent of the beds and about 60 percent of the capital investment. Rorem, who conducted the seminal survey of the industry, characterized the hospital as "a place of business" that had resulted from two trends: "(a) specialization of knowledge and skill on the part of students and practitioners in the medical field, and (b) development of types of equipment which facilitate and coordinate specialized diagnosis and treatment" [Rorem 1930, 4].

Stunted Development of the Hospital

The hospital industry had many characteristics of a business, such as sizeable capital investment, nearly 400,000 employees, and more than 2,400 for-profit institutions. Nevertheless, from an economics standpoint the hospitals more closely resembled hotels than dispensers of acute health care. Hospitals had made considerable progress from the 19th century pesthouses. However, certain elements that marked other business developments appeared to be missing from the hospital industry's maturation. Chandler [1977], a leading business historian, hypothesized that the "modern multi-unit business enterprise replaced small traditional enterprise when administrative coordination permitted greater productivity, lower costs, and higher profits than coordination by market mechanisms." The internalization or integration of market functions through the development of an enterprise's administrative capability occurred when "the visible hand of management proved to be more efficient than the invisible hand of market forces in coordinating" the activities of the industry.

Even though the hospital industry had many characteristics of a business, it was almost totally lacking in a critical element of business enterprise—entrepreneurship. In the classic sense the entrepreneur's role is to organize the production of services by providing or acquiring the risk capital, investing this capital in the full complement of resources necessary for producing the product or services, hiring qualified managers, and operating the activity as a business enterprise. The provision of acute patient care services rarely met this definition of an organized business enterprise for two principal reasons. There was no concentration of the risk-bearing responsibility and there was no centralized control of the production process within the enterprise.

First, the source of risk capital for the larger and predominantly not-for-profit public and private general hospital was so diffuse that no single person or group of individuals could legitimately claim control by virtue of bearing the entrepreneurial risk. Even judicial rulings in the 1960s holding the hospital legally responsible for patient care conducted in its facilities made little difference because the entrepreneurial risk was spread so broadly across the community. The diverse sources of capital in not-for-profit hospitals resulted in the fragmentation of the entrepreneur's role in most of these hospitals.

An exception to this general rule was Henry Ford, the extraordinary entrepreneur of the auto industry, who personally contributed all the capital for the 600-bed Henry Ford Hospital, which opened in Detroit on January 1, 1920, as a not-for-profit hospital [Sigerist 1934, 213–214]. Ford organized the production of acute care services quite unconventionally by hiring all physicians on a full-time basis at a fixed salary as a part of the acute hospital services. Earlier the legacies of two business entrepreneurs, Johns Hopkins and John D. Rockefeller, had been combined to bear the entrepreneurial risk for an innovative method of organizing medical education, biomedical research, and patient care at Johns Hopkins University and Hospital in Baltimore [Brown 1979, 132–153] and Freymann 1974, 53–59]. Again, the economic organizational innovation was the hiring of the teaching faculty, whose members also provided patient and research services, on a full-time salaried basis with a clearly identified bearer of entrepreneurial risk—in this case, a not-for- profit university corporation.

The entity must control a sufficiently large portion of the acute care production function to permit economical investment of capital and specialization of labor (the characteristics that produced the industrial revolution). It has been observed that "the remarkable aspect of the hospital organization, no matter how much the physician may be involved in policy determination, has been the organizational separation of administration of hospital personnel and physical plant from the physicians who work in [not for] the hospital" [Bugbee 1959, 897]. That is, the hospital organization did not control the production of acute care services provided within its four walls and, to that extent, is not an acute care business enterprise, but rather a medical hotel or doctor's workshop.

Even most for-profit hospitals of this period, despite the presence of a risk-bearing entrepreneur, failed to meet the condition of control over the process of production. The exceptional for-profit hospitals in 1928 that did combine responsibility and control were those institutions in which the staff physicians had invested enough capital and were a large enough group to generate a sufficient patient load to operate profitably. Virginia Mason in Seattle, Cleveland Clinic Hospital, and Doctors Hospital of New York probably were examples of institutions in which physicians had at least collectively assumed entrepreneurial control and responsibility for their organizations. Most other for-profit hospitals had little capital investment in very small facilities and were generally operated like not-for-profit hospitals with physician workshop types of control. Even the modern national for-profit or investor-owned hospital systems that were established after Medicare have basically limited their entrepreneurial activities to the management of physicians' workshops, not to the broader business of providing acute institutional patient care; i.e., medical staff control was independently maintained, and no successful efforts were made to market an integrated or comprehensive health care product.

Perhaps the most innovative acute care business organization that had been established by the end of the 1920s was an informal partnership between three prominent surgeons and five Catholic sisters with the founding of St. Mary's Hospital in Rochester, Minnesota. The three surgeons, of course, were William W. Mayo and his two sons, William J. (Will) and Charles H. Mayo. Begun in 1889 with a 45-bed hospital, the enterprise in 1929 had "no less than 386 physicians, a new building of fifteen stories with 288 examination rooms and 21 laboratories, and serving four [sic] large hospitals, which are economically independent of the clinic, but which are in charge of physicians who belong to its staff" [Sigerist 1934, 178–180]. In addition, most of the 79,000 clinic visitors in 1929 stayed in Rochester hotels until their outpatient diagnostic workups had been completed. Modern scientific medicine had become organized in a nearly perfect technical sense, and an economic enterprise had been created that truly utilized capital productively and took full advantage of specialization of labor. The Mayo family demonstrated that superb medical competence is not incompatible with great entrepreneurial skills.

In contrast the typical hospital in 1929, although still growing rapidly, did not have full-time professional management and had failed to integrate a full-time professional nursing service into its production function. Both of these resources would be added in the next decade, but a true entrepreneurial role for the hospital organizational enterprise would remain the exception. Vast improvements in the quality and sophistication of existing services were achieved. As a consequence, growth was limited to increasing the number of units produced by both individual hospitals and the hospital industry in aggregate. Not even a marketing/financing mechanism, which will be discussed next, was integrated into the hospital enterprise.

The principal reason for the failure to integrate additional functions was the lack of entrepreneurial capability in the organization. The hospital's medical staff had no market transactions except in a few institutions that had established an employment or contractual relationship with physicians. Hospitals continued to be the site for the provision of health care services, the physician's workshop, but they didn't even sell their services to the physician, only to the physician's patients. From the inception of the hospital's sale of health care services to patients, the hospital's medical staff became the paramount resource of this new business enterprise. No revenues could be earned by the hospital without a doctor's cooperation. The physician, as agent for the patient, was responsible for the direct management of patient care by writing prescriptions, ordering diagnostic tests, arranging the hospital admission, recommending surgery, and authorizing the hospital discharge.

What is surprising is that neither hospitals nor doctors, to any great extent, tried having hospitals employ physicians or having doctors purchase and operate hospitals. Either of these strategies would have resulted in the integration of hospital and medical services under the control of a single business enterprise, which could have strengthened the competitive market position of these integrated health care institutions vis-a-vis other hospitals. If those elite physicians who were trained in scientific medicine had been income maximizers, this strategy could have earned monopoly profits because of their superior knowledge in the provision of health care services.

Instead of a medical entrepreneur integrating these services, hospitals and doctors formally agreed to maintain their separate and independent roles. In fairness, it should be noted that this pattern of separation and independence has even been maintained in the most successful and largest integrated health care delivery and financing organization in the United States, the Kaiser-Permanente Medical Care Program. That program consists of three separate corporations: a medical group partnership, a hospital corporation, and the integrating health plan or insurance corporation [Somers 1971 and Carpenter 1994].

Physicians continued their traditional responsibilities for the governance of the hospital's medical staff, i.e, its organizational structure, the election of its officers, the categories of staff membership, staff appointments and delineation of professional privileges, review of patient care, and disciplinary actions concerning its staff members. Although these activities were, of course, reviewed and approved regularly by the hospital's governing authority, the physicians were a self-governing body within the hospital. Even though hospitals could charge patients for hospital services, a largely self-selected group of physicians, in effect, limited the hospital's role to that of the doctor's workshop.

DEVELOPING FINANCING AND MARKETING MECHANISMS 1930–1940

In many respects, the basic supply characteristics of America's acute health care industry were fixed by 1930. The depression stifled further organizational development of the industry and inhibited innovative forms of organization despite the addition of new private market financing and marketing mechanisms that would support the tremendous post-depression growth of the industry. With only a few relatively successful exceptions, entrepreneurship controlling sizeable quantities of resources was largely missing in the acute health care industry for the next 50 years.

Retrenchment

After nearly three decades of virtually uninterrupted prosperity and growth, except for the brief World War I period, the shock of severe depression was sharply felt by the acute health care industry. From the October 29, 1929, collapse of the stock market until the lowest point was reached in March 1933, the nation's gross national product and personal income fell by nearly one-half. Unemployment rose to nearly 13 million—a quarter of the nation's labor force. President Franklin Roosevelt's national banking holiday and his first 100 days of legislative triumphs may have helped to restore confidence in the rest of the country, but not in the medical profession or the nation's private hospitals.

By 1930 inpatient hospitalization for acute illness had become such an accepted practice that the number of patient days in general hospitals continued to rise each year, except for 1933 when the Great Depression bottomed out. However, the balance between utilization of the nation's public and private hospitals changed markedly. The depression drove patients from private hospitals, where payment for services was expected, to public hospitals, where it was not. During the 1920s private hospitals depended upon continuing expansion as the basis for financing their operations [Kingsdale 1981, 411]. Sharply falling revenues caused many smaller private hospitals to fail. Most of the smaller hospitals that failed during the 1930s were for-profit hospitals, which fell nearly one-third from 1,877 hospitals in 1928 to only 1,259 in 1940. Not-for-profit voluntary hospitals not only were larger than the proprietaries, but they had stronger financial bases, better credit ratings, and wider market appeal [Kingsdale 1981, 425].

The surviving voluntary hospitals implemented a number of internal and external innovations to meet the financial challenge of the Great Depression. Perhaps the most important internal innovation was the trustees' recognition of the need to concentrate managerial authority in the hands of professional hospital administrators. Efforts had been made since 1899 when the Association of Hospital Superintendents, which became the American Hospital Association in 1906, first met to develop professional hospital administration. Nevertheless, the local boards—often called boards of managers—still maintained a fairly tight control over the nonmedical affairs of the hospital. The financial crisis made cost control and the need for improved efficiency the bywords for stronger administrative authority residing in the hospital superintendent. During the 1930s physicians with some knowledge of business often were assigned these responsibilities until persons trained in collegiate or postgraduate programs of hospital administration became more readily available later [Kingsdale 1981, 443].

Another internal innovation was the employment of the so-called graduate nurses, who had fallen on hard times in pursuing their independent practices. Enrollment in student nursing programs had dropped in the 1930s with the apparent surplus of nurses. Thus, hospitals for the first time began to employ nurses on regular shifts in groups for both private and semiprivate patients. The grouping "allowed the hospital to charge patients extra for this service rather than include it as part of routine care" [Reverby 1979, 217] in much the same way that private duty nurses had been reimbursed previously. However, it was not until World War II, which caused substantial nursing shortages, that the practice of hiring general duty nurses and organizing a nursing team led by registered nurses became common. Specialization of other hospital employees, such as lab and x-ray technicians and physical therapists, also gained momentum during this period.

Although these internal innovations strengthened the hospital as a business enterprise, the external innovation for improving the financing and marketing of inpatient hospital services through the insurance mechanism turned financial disaster into a miraculous business success. The origins of Blue Cross will be discussed later. The important point here is that voluntary hospitals were willing to experiment with innovative financing approaches to win back their middle-class clientele from the tax-supported public hospitals.

Even before these new financing mechanisms were fully developed, the private, not-for-profit hospitals had recaptured the dominant market position by the end of the 1930s with almost two-thirds of all hospital admissions [Stevens 1989, 160]. Product improvements during the '30s were the principal source of increased demand for inpatient hospital services, especially for the not-for-profits. The use of radiology both for improved diagnostic and new therapeutic services; the development of intravenous therapies; and the first of the new "wonder" drugs, sulfanilamide, all helped boost hospital admissions. Furthermore, the growth in services for women (by 1940 56 percent of all babies were born in hospitals [Freymann 1974, 67]), and children (primarily because of tonsillectomies) between ages 5 and 9 had the second-highest hospitalization and highest surgical rate of any age group in the 1930s [Stevens 1989, 174], were responsible for making the hospital an essential element in the delivery of acute health care services.

GPs Retrocession

The hospitals' willingness to experiment during a time of financial crisis was in marked contrast to the medical profession's dogged resistance to any modification of prevailing practice. Hospitals retrenched in the '30s while the general practitioners retroceded into a bygone era. The income of the average physician fell less rapidly than that of the average American. However, there was a substantial disparity between the effect of the depression on the general practitioner (GP) and the medical specialist. Specialists on average earned 154 percent more than GPs in 1929 [Falk et al 1928, 207], and the gap widened further during the depression [Stevens 1971, 176–177]. Because of the GPs' general financial difficulties, and a rising level of animosity toward the specialist, the GPs opposed any changes in the health care delivery or financing system that would further enhance the status of the medical specialists.

When the number of scientifically educated physicians was relatively small, that elite group could serve as leaders to the profession without provoking the concerns of the majority. However, as the numbers began to balance, the great schism in knowledge could no longer be concealed. The AMA, which had been quite progressive in the first two decades of the 20th century, was geared in the third decade to represent its average membership. Although the vast gulf that Flexner had cited in 1910 between the best and the average was diminishing, it would not be fully bridged until after World War II. In the meantime, the policies that had proven successful for the profession in the first quarter of the century became gospel to medicine as the Great Depression approached. The profession's conservatism in the 1930s no doubt stemmed in large part from economic self-interest, but it was also a product of the crippling technological obsolescence that still plagued the majority of its members.

The GPs' attitudes and their numerical strength—two-thirds of all licensed physicians worked as GPs in 1931—blocked adoption of what could have been the most significant organizational reform in American medical history. The proposal for reform emerged from a five-year comprehensive study conducted by the Committee on the Costs of Medical Care (CCMC). The CCMC consisted of more than 50 prominent physicians, public health specialists, representatives of health care and educational institutions, other health care professionals, social scientists, and distinguished public representatives. This august group was supported by an outstanding research staff, many of whom played significant roles in health services research for decades, and was generously funded by eight private foundations. A comprehensive description of the existing health care delivery and financing system, with much emphasis on innovative programs, was issued in 26 separate monographs that had been prepared by the committee's research staff prior to the publication of its final report in October 1932.

The five basic recommendations adopted in the committee's final report were quite modest. It called for better organization "preferably around hospitals" of medical services by organized professional groups, the extension of all basic public health services to the entire population, the financing of medical costs through insurance and taxation, better local coordination of services, and specific recommendations for reforming professional education [CCNC 1932].

One of two separate minority reports was prepared by an eight-member physician contingent with support by the then president of the Catholic Hospital Association and dean of the St. Louis University School of Medicine. It became a manifesto for organized medicine for several decades. It attacked community medical centers as a "mass-production idea of the factory system [that will be] destructive of the social values developed by professional traditions," industrial medicine as contract practice or the corporate practice of medicine that interferes with reasonable competition and free choice of physicians, delegation of patient care responsibilities to nonmedical technicians as dangerous, private group clinics as the commercialization of medicine with the destruction of professional standards and ethics, and even voluntary insurance as the forerunner of a compulsory plan under governmental control [CCMC 1932]. Organization of medical services on any basis other than under the complete control of the medical profession and with the free choice of physician guaranteed was totally unacceptable to the authors of this minority report and subsequently to most members of organized medicine.

It did not matter that the minority report attacked concepts that had not been mandated by the majority's recommendations. Innovations for health care organization and financing that had been carried out by reputable physicians, like the Mayos, were swept aside primarily out of fear; suspicion; and, perhaps most of all, professional jealousy on the part of many GPs. The profession moved on during the 1930s to adopt reactionary positions that legitimately could be described as those of a price-discriminating monopolist who consciously restricts supply in order to earn higher income [P. Feldstein 1979, 322–337]. Regardless of the motivation for its behavior, the majority of physicians, who supported the first minority report, disrupted progress in rationally organizing health care in accordance with the principles of an efficient market.

The AMA's Blustering

A fundamental conclusion of this study is that few of these accommodations were made with any understanding or concern for their effects
on the degree of market competition that would result in the provision
and consumption of health care services in the United States. At
all stages of market development there were opportunities for some
market participants to breach these agreements and earn excess
profits, as has been demonstrated by more recent health care market
behavior. As economists are fond of noting, no producer seeks the
creation of competitive markets because competition makes producers
do what none of them would choose to do without competition—
things like reducing prices by finding lower-cost ways of producing
services or products or by developing better products that can capture
a larger share of profits in the marketplace. In most markets, producers
are not given a choice about responding to these competitive forces
because other producers are seeking to maximize their own income,
by selling the product at a lower price or higher quality to consumers
who are sensitive to product prices or quality and will seek out higher-
value producers to bring about this market competition spontane-
ously. Even when producers conspire and create cartels to fix prices
or product standards, these arrangements rarely have any long-term
stability because there is always an advantage for some producers to
sell the product with greater value than the cartel's and capture a
larger share of the profits.

If the health care marketplace behaved as other markets, one
would predict that the anticompetitive accommodations would be
eroded in the same manner as the cartel's fixed price. That is, some
producers would have been induced by profit motives to develop
more efficient delivery organization arrangements that could produce
comparable health care services at lower prices than the prices charged
for services provided by organizations constrained by the accommodations. There are at least three possible explanations for the survival
of the anticompetitive accommodations: (1) the profit motive in the
health care industry was too weak, blunted by the humanitarian service objectives of health care providers, for any producers to be motivated to defy the conventions, (2) consumers were not sufficiently
price sensitive to encourage rogue producers to gain efficiencies
through the breaking of the market conventions, or (3) there was
an unusually strong and effective enforcement mechanism for the
maintenance of the agreements.

Because there was substantial and continuing growth in the demand for health care services during the first three decades of this century, the first time in which the industry was ripe for more intense competition was the Great Depression in the 1930s when many physicians, especially general practitioners, suffered severe losses of income and private hospitals lost scores of patients to public hospitals. It is this period when lower-cost, rogue producers might have been expected to challenge the anticompetitive accommodations that constrained profit maximizing behavior. It was also a time when consumers were extremely sensitive to the price of health care services. However, the only explanation for the continuing conformance to previous accommodations and the promulgation of a new agreement on voluntary health insurance during this period that is consistent with observed behavior in the '30s is the third; the unusually strong and effective enforcer of the anticompetitive agreements was the American Medical Association and its affiliated local medical societies.

The ire of the GPs, then constituting two-thirds of all practicing physicians and an even larger majority of AMA and state and county medical societies, had been raised over the large and depression-enhanced differential in income between GPs and specialists. They had "had it" when the CCMC issued its relatively modest report advocating voluntary health insurance and group practice associated with the community hospital. The response of the AMA was vituperative in denouncing the report as a communist plot for government to take over control of medical care in the United States. The anthem of the medical profession became the organization of medical services under the complete control of the medical profession with the guarantee of free choice of physician. This emotional response was quickly translated into a series of reactionary positions by the AMA and its affiliates that could legitimately be described as those of a price-discriminating monopolist attempting to restrict the supply of physicians to earn higher income. The AMA or local medical society attacks on physicians who dared to organize unconventional health care delivery organizations or even to practice in such organizations were vicious and, subsequently, found to be illegal. No cartel in any other industry has ever found a stronger or more open enforcer than the AMA[3] became in the 1930s and early '40s.

Thus, the countervailing market forces that are normally effective in undermining anticompetitive agreements were not permitted to operate in the health care industry at a critical time in the industry's development. Although virtually all of the innovative, integrating types of health care delivery organizations that were to prosper in the last quarter of the century were extant to some degree in the '30s, their opportunity for nurturing and growth was substantially postponed by the blustering anticompetitive campaign of organized medicine.

Lost Opportunity for Entrepreneurship

The first result of the AMA's attack on competition was the rejection by voluntary hospitals of forms of hospital insurance that would have more easily led to a stronger entrepreneurial role for hospitals or insurers. Instead of pursuing those approaches, hospital associations designed a preferred insurance program that would avoid direct confrontation with organized medicine. However, it must be emphasized that following even that course in the early 1930s was no simple matter. The idea of health insurance had been rejected earlier by the insurance industry experts in the belief that health care was not an insurable risk [MacIntyre 1962, 124].

Prepayment and various forms of employee or association health benefits were not new ideas. The CCMC research monographs had identified several successful approaches. Employers had formed associations to contract with physician groups for comprehensive health care services; a private clinic group, also owning a hospital, would contract with employers or individuals for these services; and a large group of employees would form physician and hospital associations to provide care to association members [Falk et al 1928, 485].

In the late 1920s individual hospitals, the most famous of which was the Baylor Hospital prepayment plan for Dallas school teachers, offered to various employee groups or associations a specific number of days of hospital care per year in exchange for an annual and monthly prepayment fee.[4] A variation of this plan involved a proprietary organization performing the promotion, selling, collection, and administrative functions for either a single hospital or groups of hospitals.

Of those options that had been tried by the early 1930s, the comprehensive prepayment arrangements offered the greatest opportunity for an entrepreneur to develop an integrated acute health care delivery system with the rational investment of capital and a systematic basis for the specialization of labor. The least integration of the delivery system would result from the marketing of prepayment on a cooperative basis by groups of hospitals in a geographic area. Single-hospital prepayment plans, such as Baylor's, concentrated the risk on that hospital and restricted the subscriber's choice of physician to those having appointments on that hospital's medical staff. The individual hospital plans were unacceptable to organized medicine because such plans violated the profession's freedom of choice principle. However as Kingsdale [1981, 494] speculates, these programs might well have led to hospital-based group practice health maintenance organizations had they been encouraged to spread in the 1930s.

Instead of competitive plans, prepayment for hospital care was established on a cooperative group basis by an action of the American Hospital Association (AHA) in 1933. Michael Davis and Rufus Rorem, both of whom had been on the research staff of the CCMC and had the support of the Julius Rosenwald Fund, met with the AHA officers to formulate a proposal for the voluntary financing of hospital care. That proposal was approved by the AHA Board of Trustees in February over the objections of the American Medical Association (AMA). Rorem was immediately loaned to the AHA by the Rosenwald Fund and his first assignment was to prepare a list of essential criteria for an acceptable group hospitalization plan, which was approved in April.

These criteria emphasized the not-for-profit, public welfare nature of the voluntary insurance program and the need for professional and public interest representation on the plan governing boards. They stressed the importance of economic and actuarial soundness in the insurance operations, which were to be promoted in a dignified, noncommercial manner. But most important, in deference to the American Medical Association, the plans were to be structured to guarantee that the insureds would have "free choice of physician and hospital" and that the benefits would be limited to hospital services, i.e., physician and surgeon services had to be separated from the hospital benefits [Davis 1955, 216–217].

In January 1933 the first hospital cooperative prepayment plan was organized in Essex County, New Jersey, along the lines of the essentials through a local hospital council. Its primary objective was to serve as the hospitals' collection agency because it was believed that collecting on the patients' receivables could be made less onerous by organizing patient financing on a prepayment rather than postpayment basis [Van Dyk 1933]. The first rudimentary actuarial studies using CCMC data served as the basis for establishing prepayment rates by observing that hospital utilization was approximately 700 to 800 admissions per 10,000 population and that average length of stay per admission was 10 or 11 days. Six months later a plan was started in Minnesota using for the first time a Blue Cross symbol [Anderson 1975, 35–37]. Three more plans were launched in 1933, and Blue Cross was off and running. By the end of 1940 there were 56 plans with a total enrollment of more than six million. Enabling legislation had been also approved in 40 states to exempt non-profit Blue Cross plans from the incorporation and reserve requirements imposed on insurance companies as well as from taxes on earned income [The Somers 1961, 294], and the AHA had developed standards for accrediting Blue Cross plans.

The initial success of prepayment health insurance led commercial insurance companies to reconsider and enter this new insurance market. However, the insurance actuaries had several concerns that led to differences in the type of coverage offered. Instead of writing their hospital coverage in terms of service benefits generally used by the Blue Cross plans, commercial carriers wrote benefits in terms of a fixed-dollar amount, an indemnity basis, for each day of hospitalization. They established their rates according to the insured group's actual experience instead of the community rating approach of Blue Cross.

These differences reflected the actuaries' belief that the hazard or risk being insured needed to be defined in ways consistent with "traditional insurance concepts of limited liability" [MacIntyre, 1962, 124]. The actuaries were concerned that first-dollar service benefits would cause the insureds to increase their utilization of health care services and that higher-risk individuals were more likely to purchase health insurance than healthier persons. Both of these concerns were validated by subsequent events in the postwar period.

By the end of 1940 more than three and one-half million persons had acquired commercial health insurance coverage. In addition, more than two million others were enrolled in employment programs or in comprehensive group practice arrangements. Despite the vigorous and occasionally illegal opposition of organized medicine, physician-initiated programs, such as the Ross-Loos Clinic in Los Angeles, and medical cooperatives, like the one established in Elk City, Oklahoma, by Dr. Michael Shadid, were organized and began to grow. Nevertheless in the next phase of development it was the entry of commercial carriers writing a health insurance product in competition with the

Blue Cross prepayment model that had the more signficant effect on the health care service market.

By the end of 1940 health insurance even included medical or surgical coverage for some five million persons. The American College of Surgeons had broken with the AMA by endorsing the AHA's voluntary hospital insurance in 1933 and later supported coverage for inhospital physician services. The state medical societies in California and in Michigan also broke with the AMA and formed medical service plans in 1939 that later became the Blue Shield plans. The AMA finally endorsed the principle of medical service plans in 1943 and developed its own Blue Shield approval program in 1946.

The schism between hospital-based specialists, who supported health insurance, and the general practitioners, who opposed it, caused health insurance coverage to be limited to those services provided within the hospital. This limitation encouraged physicians to retain services within the hospital that, from a technical standpoint, probably could have been provided on an outpatient basis much sooner than actually occurred. Patients wanted the services to be covered by insurance, and their doctors obliged them by performing the services in the hospital.

Organized medicine's opposition may have slowed, and certainly altered, the pattern of health insurance growth, but it could not prevent the development of needed financing mechanisms for the vast middle-class clientele. These programs reflected the basic willingness of Americans to spread the risk of costly hospitalization. The premium costs were paid by the consumers themselves even though many of the policies were purchased at their places of employment to reduce the administrative costs of the programs. Blue Cross had tried to insist on employer administration of the programs to reduce cost and enhance sales. This practice became one of the key factors in the success of Blue Cross and Blue Shield and subsequently helped to overcome the commercial insurance carriers objections to writing health insurance.

These insurance programs and the general business recovery caused occupancy rates in voluntary not-for-profit hospitals in 1940 to exceed 70 percent, which was significantly higher than the predepression occupancy levels. Just as dispersion of risk through communitywide fund raising had permitted acute care hospitals to acquire capital earlier, insurance programs for individual consumers based on this same principle had enabled voluntary hospitals to weather their most severe financial crisis. However, broad community owner-ship of these institutions with its dispersion of risk would also continue to limit the role of the entrepreneur in organizing the acute health care industry.

POISED FOR GROWTH

In 1940 the health care industry had just completed a decade in which some real growth had been achieved while the rest of the economy had declined. However, the resource constraints resulting from America's preparations for fighting World War II postponed the industry's growth phase from beginning in earnest until the war's conclusion. Except for dire needs for capital for plant and equipment whose re-placement and expansion had been delayed by the Great Depression, the industry was in an excellent position for the commencement of a long period of sustained growth.

Although scientific medicine and its organized site for care, the hospital, had made considerable progress in improving its product and developing a marketing/financing mechanism, this 40-year gestation period was not only considerably longer than the introductory periods experienced by other industries, but certain competitive elements in the makeup of the industry were missing that had been experienced in the market development of others. The developmental precedent had been established for doctors and hospitals to reach accommoda-tion instead of competition in the health care marketplace. Other market participants would soon be engulfed by the spirit of accommo-dation that had been achieved.

3

The Imprinting of Scientific Medicine on America, 1941–1965

In the 25 years from 1941 to 1965 the health care industry, led by the hospital, became one of the fastest growing sectors in the American economy. The growth in scientific medicine was financed by private health insurance coupled with generous federal subsidies for research and for human and facilities resources development, but the real source of growth stemmed from the imprinting of the American consumer with the value of scientific medicine. Health care spending would rise from 4.1 percent of gross national product in 1940 to nearly 6 percent in 1965. However, this initial growth phase for health care was simply the opening act in a surrealistic play that established an almost frictionless growth environment, unlike any other market in the U.S. economy. The economic law of supply and demand for determining resource allocation was replaced by a supplier(provider)-dominated market almost totally devoid of the normal competitive pressures.

Without price competition among suppliers, an inertia set in that immobilized the economic entities in the health care marketplace in their prewar configurations. Despite unfavorable court rulings striking down the most strident AMA boycotts of group practice, the prewar anticompetitive agreements became entrenched as consumers, labor unions, and the federal government all worked to make employer-sponsored first-dollar health insurance programs part of the American dream. As a consequence, the 1930s trends toward increased physician specialization and inpatient hospital utilization continued unabated. Instead of unleashing competitive forces that would create delivery system alternatives to the hospital-physician alliance, this period proved pivotal in extending that alliance well beyond the best interests of either party and certainly to the detriment of healthy market development.

PERFECT TIMING FOR GROWTH

Timing proved to be everything in understanding American consumers' attitudes toward health insurance and their insurance "buying" habits. In fact, the strength and rigidity of American consumers' insurance purchasing behavior almost suggests that it was learned by imprinting, the learning process that occurs early in the development of a social animal in which a specific behavior pattern becomes fixed by observing and emulating a role model.

American consumers were certainly in their first generation of buying health insurance when wartime wage and price controls encouraged employers, in competing for workers, to provide "free" health insurance coverage as an employee fringe benefit. Prior to the war, a small, but growing, group of consumers had willingly paid their own insurance premiums, asking only that employers serve as their collection agent to reduce administrative expenses. After World War II labor unions fought to institutionalize the health insurance benefit in their negotiations with large industrial employers. Their efforts were assisted by a series of favorable administrative and judicial rulings, and the popularity of their campaign was enhanced by the coincidental release of the recently discovered "wonder drugs," antibiotics that had the most salutory impact on health of any of the products of scientific medicine.

Making Health Care a Fringe Benefit

The wartime period was relatively uneventful in the development of the delivery component of the health care industry.[5] The civilian population coped with a host of shortages, including resources for the provision of medical care. With so many qualified physicians and nurses serving military personnel, both human and capital resources for civilian health care services were severely constrained. The only significant delivery organization change was the integration of nursing into hospital employment during this period. The backlog of needed equipment and hospital facilities continued to grow from the 1930s.

Despite the shortage of resources, this period marked an important turning point in the industry's ability to finance both its capital and operating expenditures. Private health insurance was given standing in collective bargaining, along with other fringe benefits, which guaranteed its successful marketing in the postwar economy. The decision to treat employee fringe benefits differently than cash wages was based initially on the need to make wartime wage and price controls more palatable. Mandatory price controls had been imposed in 1942 with a voluntary wage stabilization program to combat inflation generated by the substantial increase in disposable income while the production of consumer goods was being severely curtailed. Wage controls became mandatory in April 1943 but were accompanied by the "institution and liberalization of fringe benefits such as vacations, holidays, or health and welfare plans" [Bloom and Northrup 1955, 478]. Unions experienced their greatest growth in membership from 3.9 million in 1935 to 15 million in 1946, and they obviously were encouraged to bargain for these largely uncontrolled nonwage benefits.

After the war, the doors to the U.S. treasury were permanently opened to finance a substantial portion of employees' health insurance premiums. In 1947 the National Labor Relations Board, later sustained by the U.S. Supreme Court, ruled "that employer contributions to insurance and pension plans were wages and therefore subject to collective bargaining" [MacIntyre 1962, 146–147]. The effect of this ruling "not only required employers to negotiate [these benefits] . . . when requested to do so but also prohibited employers from changing existing plans without consulting the legally certified bargaining agent representing their employees" [Becker 1955, 20–21, with explanation that health insurance was explicitly recognized in 1948]. The tax laws, which grew in importance as rates rose during this period, were also "liberalized" to exclude employer contributions for qualified fringe benefits from the employees' taxable income.

As a part of the fringe benefit package the market for private health insurance was given a tremendous boost by the growth of union membership, the inclusion of fringes as a central element in the collective bargaining arena, and the favorable tax treatment for fringe benefits. These three factors, plus the inherent popularity of health insurance, led to more than a tenfold increase in the number of persons enrolled in hospital insurance programs by the end of the 1950s. Enrollments rose from less than 10 million in 1940 to nearly

130 million, or about 72 percent of the population. In addition, almost two-thirds of the population had insurance coverage providing surgical benefits, and nearly one-half had regular medical coverage. Although the growing strength of labor unions and the favorable tax laws encouraged full employer contributions for health insurance premiums, only "26 percent of the families with group hospital insurance in 1958 had all of their premiums paid by the employer; 44 percent had some paid; [and] 17 percent paid the entire premium themselves" [The Somers 1961, 228]. Most Americans still had a significant financial stake in the cost of health insurance premiums, but they were overwhelmingly choosing to obtain coverage regardless of who paid.

The Age of Antibiotics

Table 3.1 summarizes the death rates in the United States for the first six decades in the 20th century. The availability of employer-sponsored health insurance fringe benefits coincided with the greatest contribution of the branch of medical science stemming from Pasteur's germ theory. Beginning in 1928 with Fleming's discovery of penicillin and followed by sulfa in the 1930s, a whole series of antibiotic drugs were developed that almost totally eradicated the most serious infectious diseases. The widespread distribution of these drugs after World War II caused a dramatic reduction in the nation's age-adjusted death rate (as the population grows older, the death rate rises and this adjustment adjusts for the aging of the population). Freymann [1974,

TABLE 3.1   U.S. Mortality in the 20th Century
For Selected Years between 1900–1960

Year	Age-Adjusted Death Rate per 1,000	Percent Decrease
1900	17.8	—
1910	15.8	11.2
1920	14.3	10.1
1930	12.5	12.0
1940	10.8	13.6
1950	8.4	22.2
1960	7.6	9.5

Source: National Centers for Health Statistics and Health Services Research [1977].

13] defines the precise period of the age of antibiotics in the United States as occurring from 1936 to 1954 when the death rate declined at an annual rate of 1.5 percent, and he notes that "every one of the industrialized countries went through this same experience at about the same time."

Spurred by the manufacture of antibiotics and other new prescription drugs, such as tranquilizers, the drug industry experienced a tenfold growth in sales in the 30 years since 1929. Prescription drugs increased from 50 percent of total drug sales in the 1930s to nearly 80 percent in 1960, and direct consumer expenditures for drugs accounted for just over 20 percent of the nation's total health care expenditures in the early 1950s. Physicians armed with "the new 'wonder drugs', vaccines, and insecticides against acute communicable diseases [were able to nearly eliminate] pneumonia, scarlet fever, streptococcal infection, diphtheria, tuberculosis, whooping cough, paralytic polio, and other former 'killers'" [The Somers 1961, 92].

The benefits of scientific medicine were now tangible for all to see and experience. With typical American optimism, expectations rose to even greater heights as nonbacterial illnesses and diseases were viewed as the next battle to be fought and won by laboratory sciences and technology.

The Benevolence of Government

Although the federal government had done relatively little in health care prior to World War II,[6] no player in the health care marketplace was more enthusiastic than the Congress in supporting scientific medicine. The principal new purpose for federal legislative activity during this period was to direct federal largesse to increase the nation's health research capabilities through the expansion of the National Institutes of Health. The Public Health Act of 1944 provided for research grants to nonfederal entities. Health care professionals were supported, beginning in 1941 with the Nurse Training Act to increase the supply of nurses available to the armed services. Health facilities also benefitted, starting with a priority for subsidizing the construction of rural hospitals through the Hospital Survey and Construction Act in 1946 (Hill-Burton) and later chronic hospitals, rehabilitation facilities, nursing homes, and research facilities. Although virtually every category of illness and type of health care or research facility had been identified for federal government support by 1960, the funds really began to flow after Kennedy's inauguration; through President Lyndon's Johnson's Great Society program; and, because of strong congressional support, until the mid-1970s.

The first major program of federal benevolence after World War II was well designed; quite effective in improving access to health care; and, as a result, politically popular. During the 1930s and the war hospitals had been unable to invest in new construction, renovation, or repair of facilities; and communities without hospital facilities were unable to build them. This shortage had been recognized in 1941 with approval of the Lanham Act, which provided for the building of hospital facilities in areas that were growing because of industrial expansion for defense production.

Partnerships between the hospital industry and the U.S. Public Health Service and between federal and state health departments were the modus operandi for the 1946 Hill-Burton Act. Initially, state health departments gathered data on existing hospital beds for different population density areas and identified plans for meeting bed shortages for these areas. When grants, which were to finance up to 15 percent of the construction of new short-term general hospitals, were authorized in 1949 priority was given to poorer states and to shortage areas, generally rural communities, within those states. Thus, the program followed a rational process for defining need and used the federal dollars to encourage local fund-raising activities for the major cost of the new hospitals—truly an effective partnership between the federal government and local communities.

Periodically, Congress revised the program's priorities for the type of health care facility requiring subsidization. In 1954 outpatient diagnostic and treatment centers and hospitals for the chronically ill and rehabilitation were made eligible, in 1964 modernization of existing facilities became eligible, and in 1970 a loan guarantee program was added as a partial substitute for grants.

In their 1974 study of the Hill-Burton program, Judith and Lester Lave concluded that "the program did serve to increase the number of both short-term beds and total beds per thousand, an effect that would not have taken place to the extent it did in the program's absence . . . did not . . . lower occupancy rates [across states and] it probably affected the distribution of physicians" [The Laves 1974]. The Laves' biggest complaint about the program was Congress' unwillingness to terminate it in 1973 as President Nixon recommended. Like the old soldier, the program wouldn't die, but neither would it fade away.

Although federal support for biomedical research may have been as politically popular as the support for hospital construction, neither the concept nor the operation of the federal grant program for research followed the principles of effective government that marked the Hill-Burton program. In 1944 the National Institutes of Health allocated $150,000 for research grants to nonfederal agencies out of a total budget of $2.5 million. From this modest beginning, a cabal[7] consisting of Mrs. Mary Lasker and her friend, Mrs. Florence Mahoney; Senator Lister Hill of Alabama; Congressman John E. Fogarty of Rhode Island; and Dr. James A. Shannon, who later became director of NIH, built "the NIH in two decades into the largest, richest, and most powerful research agency the world had ever seen" [Freymann 1974, 84]. The NIH's budget rose to $80 million in 1950, $430 million in 1960, and reached the billion dollar mark in 1965—400 times the original appropriation in just over 20 years, an annual growth rate of 33 percent.

Even under the most structured, planned circumstances, spending funds wisely at that rate of growth is a very difficult managerial problem. Unlike the Hill-Burton program, there was no preestablished strategy or goals for the expenditure of these funds even though NIH conducted detailed peer-review evaluations of specific grant proposals. The public was awestruck by the success of the "wonder drugs" in eradicating infectious diseases, and Congress couldn't appropriate enough funds for biomedical research. For 14 consecutive years from 1953 to 1966 the congressional appropriations for NIH exceeded the administration's budgetary requests, and during this period five new NIH institutes were established.

It was clearly the intent of Congress that some of these research appropriations were to be used for general support of the nation's medical schools because Congress was unwilling to approve direct support for medical education over the vigorous objections of the American Medical Association. It is doubtful, however, that either Mary Lasker or Congress would have been willing to allocate more than 60 percent of the funds to general support of medical education, as some expert observers believe actually occurred [Freymann 1974, 88].

STIFLING HEALTH CARE COMPETITION

The 1930s anticompetitive agreements between doctors and hospitals now became locked in place by the supportive behavior of the federal government during and after World War II. Except for antitrust prosecution of AMA's most outlandish boycotts to block competition, the federal government during this period consistently acted in ways that either sanctified or aggrandized hospital-doctor agreements. First, in a series of judical and administrative decisions employer-provided first-dollar health insurance benefits were institutionalized as a part of collective bargaining in U.S. labor markets. Then, both congressmen and presidents, who wanted to assist their constituents in obtaining the politically-popular fruits of medical science, extended government largess to the fiscal needs of the rapidly developing health care industry. Instead of trying to aid constructively in the development of the industry, as the Hill-Burton program had done by planning for health facility needs before making federal grants, most federal programs simply threw money at health care organizations in an unplanned manner that further strengthened the position of the advocates of scientific medicine. Again, the efforts of the AMA, in simply opposing federal assistance for medical education, worked against the interests of primary care physicians and helped advocates of scientific medicine and basic sciences against the interests of community medicine by having medical school grants channeled through science departments.

Commercial insurance carriers entered the health insurance market in a big way during and after World War II because the employer sponsorship of health insurance, which ensured that all members of the employment group were covered, overcame one of actuaries objections to writing health risks—self-selection and the consequent higher proportion of adverse risks that would have had to be insured. Although the entry of commercial insurance carriers nominally increased competition in the health insurance market, it did not assist in developing competition between different types of health care delivery organizations. It was the lack of delivery organization competition coupled with the resulting first or low dollar health insurance coverage that substantially raised future health care costs. The historical accident of wage controls luring employers into providing their employees during World War II with "free" health insurance coverage simply added fuel to the already inflationary health care marketplace.

Paradoxically, at this time the American Medical Association did not act in the best economic interest of its members, who were largely general practitioners, for it opposed the efforts to create voluntary health insurance and "successfully" restricted its benefits to hospital-related services. Specialization in scientific medicine as well as the interest of hospitals thus gained greater strength in the health care marketplace, and future health care costs were to be inflated further.

Competition Among Health Insurers

If marketing success is measured in terms of increased expenditures for a product, then the marketing of private health insurance since its inception in the late 1920s and early 1930s must be ranked as the greatest marketing achievment of this century. During this period expenditures for private health insurance grew from almost nothing to more than $216 billion in 1990, almost 4 percent of America's gross national product. The key marketing strategy was the Blue Cross decision in the '30s to link the sale of hospital insurance with the employment relationship, which was done primarily to reduce administrative and sales costs. However inadvertent, this strategy, augmented unintentionally by the federal government, resulted in a competition between insurers that outperformed any Madison Avenue sales campaign ever undertaken.

If the battle for fringes was fought by labor and management negotiators aided and abetted by federal regulators, the battle over health insurance fringes was fought principally by Blue Cross/Blue Shield and private insurance companies. The primary tactic was competition involving the design and pricing of health insurance benefits. Administrative efficiency and consumer convenience were secondary issues.

The two competitors began marketing benefits designed in accordance with their origins. Blue Cross plans, supported by the AHA and state hospital associations, were developed as public service organizations to provide subscribers with hospital services, and minimum coverage was measured by the Blue Cross plan's assuming at least 75 percent of the subscriber's liability regardless of the total dollar amount of the hospital bill, which was typically interpreted as full coverage for semi-private room accommodations. Insurance companies, on the other hand, had been accustomed to limiting their liabilities to fixed dollar amounts that could be more easily determined actuarially like the casualty and disability losses insurance companies traditionally insured. Thus, private health insurers initially limited their benefit design to fixed dollar or indemnity coverage.

During the postwar competition between the Blues and the commercials for employee group business the commercials tended to offer a more service benefit type of package while the Blues incorporated some limited indemnity benefits into an otherwise service benefit package.

In 1948, the private carriers also began to market major medical benefits, which were a compromise between the two types of benefit structures. Major medical plans were to assume a fixed percentage of the enrollee's medical bill after the enrollee had exhausted the basic benefits in the coverage or the payment of a first-dollar deductible of a specified amount and then a proportional sharing of health care costs beyond that amount. Virtually all major medical policies had some established limit on the total liability of the insurance company. Major medical coverage, especially as a supplement to basic group insurance, became quite popular. By the end of the 1950s "the enrollment figure exceeded 20 million, with slightly less than 14 million covered by supplemental plans and about 6.5 million covered by comprehensive plans" [MacIntyre 1962, 61]. With major medical enrollment exceeding 20 percent of the group business, this new form of coverage was helpful to commercial carriers in their competition with Blue Cross and Blue Shield plans.

One advantage that the Blues were able to exploit through their hospital sponsorship was to develop direct contractual relationships with these hospitals and to negotiate cost-based reimbursement contracts. Direct contractual relationships made it possible for Blue Cross subscribers to pay their hospital bills by having the charges, or at least Blue Cross' share, sent directly to the Blue Cross plan. Beneficiaries of commercial carriers had to pay the hospital and then submit the paid bills to the private health insurance company for reimbursement.

Cost-based reimbursement contracts were first negotiated between a Blue Cross plan and hospitals in 1938 in northeast Ohio. Since both Blue Cross and hospitals in the area were nonprofit organizations, it was argued that hospitals should only charge these "prepayment" patients the actual cost of care so that these patients would not be subsidizing the cost of other patients' care [Becker 1955, 305–306].

In many instances, the development of retrospective cost-based reimbursement formulas for determining the price of care for Blue Cross patients resulted in a price advantage for the Blues in their competition with commercial insurance carriers. As noted earlier, the precedent of the Blue Cross cost basis of payment was also sought for the federal government's purchase of hospital services.

The market competition also influenced the administrative practices and organizational structure of the competing entities. Blue Cross and Blue Shield had developed as regional organizations with decentralized decision making and control. Most of the large commercial firms were national entities with strong centralized control. In order to compete with these firms for national contracts with employers that had operations scattered over several states, Blue Cross and Blue Shield had to create an administrative structure that would permit cooperation among several plans. Efforts were made in 1948 to form a joint national commission of Blue Cross and Blue Shield plans, but the American Medical Association refused to support the joint venture [Anderson 1975, chapter 7].

In the early 1950s agreements were reached that permitted the joint marketing of hospital (Blue Cross) and medical (Blue Shield) benefits nationally. Both organizations also developed through their respective national commissions an interplan service benefit bank; an interplan transfer agreement; and other arrangements, including a national advertising program, to write and efficiently administer national accounts [Anderson 1975, chapter 8].

However, the major turning point in the development of the health insurance market was the commercial companies' method of calculating premiums. The commercial rates reflected the actual health care cost experience of the firm purchasing the insurance. On the other hand, Blue Cross was philosophically committed to a community rating, which averaged the health care costs across the entire area's insured population. Although community rating was simpler to administer, commercial carriers had a competitive advantage because writing insurance for groups with lower cost experience would justify lower rates than the community average. Such groups chose commercial coverage to reduce their premiums or increase benefits. The effect on the Blue's community rates for the remaining population was to increase the difference in premium rates even more. Eventually the Blues were forced to abandon their philosophy and determine rates on each group's own health care cost experience.

Once both types of insurers had adopted experience rating, there ceased to be any real insurance function in the health care market. The carriers were no longer at risk, but only provided a budgeting mechanism for employers. As Daniel Pettengill of Aetna described the effect of experience rating, "At the end of each year, the insurer reassesses and says 'Next year the budget's got to be bigger. So if you want the same benefits, Mr. Employer or Mr. Union, you have to pay more'" [Weeks and Berman 1985]. The dominant insurance mechanism became a very efficient money changer by converting employer/employee premium dollars into hospital/physician revenues without exercising any restraint on health care costs.

By the end of the 1950s, both Blue Cross/Blue Shield and the commercial carriers had enrolled over 50 million in group hospital insurance, and the private carriers had written hospital coverage for an additional 30 million individuals. The basic design of the private market's health insurance benefit package was based on the medical profession's hallowed principles of the patient's freedom to choose a personal physician and a fee-for-service system of provider payment. The anticompetitive agreements between doctors and hospitals now had a marketing-financing mechanism that passed along their costs to employers who more and more frequently gave their employees "free" first-dollar health insurance coverage.

Alternative Financing Systems

Nevertheless, a number of innovative systems were developed during this period. The most successful, and subsequently the largest, was organized by another great business entrepreneur, Henry J. Kaiser, whose industrial enterprises have grown into a multibillion dollar a year operation. In 1942 Kaiser, assisted by Dr. Sidney Garfield, created the Kaiser Health Plan, a hospital corporation, and a medical group practice partnership to provide comprehensive medical and hospital services to 90,000 Kaiser shipyard employees in the San Francisco-Oakland metropolitan area. The organization was based on Dr. Garfield's experience in providing medical services through a multispecialty group practice to Kaiser employees engaged in the construction of the Grand Coulee Dam in a remote region of Washington state. After the war, the Kaiser Health Plan opened its enrollment to the general population. The comprehensive prepayment arrangement in which the plan "undertakes not only to pay for medical and related services but also to assure that they will be available and actually rendered" [Fleming 1971, 25] shattered both of the medical profession's hallowed principles by limiting patient choice to the medical group practice and by paying physicians on a capitation basis—an annual fee per registrant for total medical services. By the end of the '50s Kaiser had moved into the Portland, Los Angeles, and Hawaiian markets through a carefully controlled and self-financed program of growth.

The closed panel group practice system of medical care delivery coupled with prepayment and capitation, or salaried physician remuneration, was replicated in other locales during the 1940s and 1950s. None of the other major alternative delivery systems centralized entrepreneurial risk and responsibility in quite the way the Kaiser system concentrated the entrepreneurial role. Most of the other systems were organized through consumer or employee groups. For example, the Group Health Cooperative of Puget Sound, founded in 1947 when a group of families purchased a small hospital and organized a multispecialty group practice; the Health Insurance Plan of Greater New York, also founded in 1947 "with the primary purpose of providing prepaid medical care to employees of the City of New York" [The Somers 1961, 351]; the Group Health Association of Washington, started in 1937 by employees of the Federal Home Owners Loan Corporation, but was subjected to such harassment by the District of Columbia Medical Society that successful operation was not achieved until it obtained judicial relief from the U.S. Supreme Court in 1943; some 50 union-organized health care programs, pioneered by the International Ladies Garment Workers Union in 1913; and most dramatically exemplified by the United Mine Workers program in 1948.

Despite the isolated successes of many of these independent financing and health care delivery organizations, they had captured less than 4 percent of the health insurance market by the end of the 1950s. The resistance of organized medicine to any tampering with the freedom of choice and fee-for-service principles was a significant impediment to the growth of these innovative alternatives. The tactics of the local medical societies in discouraging physician involvement included moral suasion through policy pronouncements attacking "contract medicine," direct economic competition through the operations of Blue Shield medical insurance plans, and expulsion of the contract physicians from the local medical society. This last tactic could be especially devastating to the development of alternative delivery systems if local hospitals required medical society membership as a condition for hospital staff memberships and privileges. This practice was subsequently found to violate provisions of the Sherman Antitrust Act in the landmark case of American Medical Association v. United States 317 U.S. 519 (1943) involving the Group Health Association of Washington. During the 1940s and 1950s a number of antitrust suits redressed grievances stemming from illegal harassment by medical societies of group practices and alternative delivery organizations. For example, the Group Health Cooperative of Puget Sound in 1951 resorted to litigation to stop the King County Medical Society from boycotting its member physicians, and the Community Hospital-Clinic of Elk City, Oklahoma, obtained an out-of-court settlement of $300,000 for "restraint of trade" violations by the local medical society in 1952 [The Somers 1961, 348–349; also see Kessel [1958] and Goldberg and Greenberg 1978].

Even without the illegal harassment of medical societies, there is doubt that these alternative delivery organizations could have attained a fair market test. More and more American consumers, as "free" first-dollar health insurance coverage grew, had no incentive to abandon their freedom of choice of physician and restrict their medicial care to a closed group of physicians. Consequently, even the most ideologically committed of organized labor chose to negotiate for increased health insurance coverage instead of pursuing the course charted by the United Mine Workers in establishing its own health care delivery system. The steelworkers in a 1959 strike originally sought a UMW-type medical program but later settled within the Blue Cross/Blue Shield framework. Even the ideologically committed United Auto Workers, which had continued to operate an independent health plan in Detroit, bargained for a basic Blue Cross and Blue Shield set of benefits, but also utilized alternative delivery mechanisms where available as a part of its health fringe benefit [The Somers 1961, 234–238].

Postwar Medical Practice

The war's intrusion after a decade of depression did not alter the course of medical practice in the United States. Although Stevens [1971, 267] has speculated that "a more Machiavellian profession might have seized the opportunity inherent in the disruptions of World War II to rebuild general practice, to redefine general-specialist relations, to examine the emerging role of the hospital" the dominant patterns of increased specialization and solo practice continued in the postwar era.

Specialization is, of course, essential to coping with the ever expanding body of medical knowledge, for it was becoming humanly impossible to encompass the encyclopedia of medical knowledge [Freymann 1974, 65]. Postwar prosperity and public subsidy of graduate medical education financed the returning physician's graduate education in a specialized area of medical practice. Once the system of graduate education was developed to accommodate the rush of returning GIs, residency training became a permanent fixture in physician education. The key ruling was made by the Veterans Administration in 1945 that "payment of tuition and living allowances could be made to hospitals and to physicians taking graduate training in acceptable hospitals [Stevens 1971, 299] as part of the GI bill, the Serviceman's Readjustment Act of 1944. Postwar medical school graduates came to accept the residency as a routine part of their medical education. In fact, the expanded capacity of the U.S. residency program developed during this period later served to attract increasingly larger numbers of foreign medical school graduates to America.

After World War II, the medical specialist became the standard in American medicine and not a technocratic elite as it had been prior to the war. By 1960 full-time specialist practice constituted more than one-half of all medical practices, rising from less than one-quarter of all practices in 1940. Further, the specialists were no longer concentrated in large urban settings surrounding major medical school centers. Many full-time specialists had migrated to suburban and smaller city practices. Although medical schools had grown into scientific and research enclaves with almost complete independence from their parent universities, the community hospital through its residency programs had also become an attractive site for specialty practice. "By 1960, internships and residencies were offered in 1,400 hospitals which contained among them almost half of the hospital beds in the country" [Stevens 1971, 380].

Despite the fact that internal medicine and pediatrics were two of the fastest growing specialties, the absolute number and the ratio of family physicians to the population fell substantially during the postwar period [Fein 1967, 71–72]. The principal cause, as Table 3.2 reports, was the retirement from practice of such large numbers of general practitioners during this period, including the last of the pre-

TABLE 3.2   Decline of GP AND Family Physicians as Percentage of Total Practicing Physicians in Selected Years between 1940–1965

Type of Practice	1940	1949	1957	1965
Pediatrics	2,222	3,787	5,876	9,726
Int. Medicine	5,892	10,923	14,654	22,432
Gen. Practice	109,272	95,526	81,443	65,951
Primary Care	117,386	110,236	101,973	98,109
% of Total	67.0%	54.8%	45.0%	37.2%
Other Practices	57,777	91,041	124,652	164,217
Total Practicing	175,153	201,277	226,625	262,326

Source: Fein [1967, p. 72], who made the calculations from data reported in U.S. Public Health Service, *Health Resources Statistics*, 1965 with the 1965 total number of practicing physicians estimated by extrapolation.

Flexner trained physicians. The United States had finally achieved Flexner's dream, and the average American doctor had "been transformed . . . from an incompetent physician, whose strength lay in the 'bedside manner' of his mystique, to a specialist internist, surgeon, or endocrinologist . . . American doctors [were] among the best trained, perhaps the best trained technological physicians in the world" [Stevens 1971, 374]. In addition to the concern that America may have produced too many surgical specialists, who had risen from about 10 percent to more than 25 percent of all physicians by 1960, it was becoming increasingly difficult to find a family physician who made house calls. In 1931, 40 percent of physician visits occurred in the patient's home. House calls accounted for only 2 percent of physician visits by the mid 1960s [Freymann 1974, 68].

The advances in pharmacology and other related sciences during this period, coupled with the geographical spread of specialty practice, should have challenged the structure and economics of medical practice. However, the organization and economic basis of practice remained almost exclusively solo and fee-for-service. The American Medical Association's 1959 survey of medical groups reported that 13,009 physicians were engaged in full-time (11,620) or part-time (1,389) group practice [AMA 1968]. This represented just over 6 percent of all practicing physicians. In 1959 the AMA's survey did not even break out data on multispecialty groups.

Although solo practice for the generalist may have had some logical basis, the fragmentation of medical knowledge into specialty areas and the rapidity with which new information became available certainly should have called for a reassessment of Will Mayo's 50-year old admonition to the profession. Mayo in 1910 had said:

> "As we men of medicine grow in learning, we more justly appreciate our dependence upon each other . . . . It has become necessary to develop medicine as a cooperative science; the clinician, the specialist and the laboratory workers uniting for the good of the patient, each assisting in the elucidation of the problem at hand, and each dependent upon the other for support . . . . Individualism in medicine can no longer exist." [Clapesattle 1954, 315–316]

Mayo's dream for the integration of specialized medical skills was still not to be realized in general, at least not in the physician's office practice.

The federal government's financing of medical schools under the guise of research grants distorted the political power of different faculty specialties within the schools, and laboratory scientists became the schools' rainmakers. Nearly a generation of medical school students were attracted to postgraduate research instead of honing their clinical or caring skills. A huge booster shot had been given to strengthen the strain of scientism within the medical profession without any conscious consideration of how such a policy would affect the future of health care in the United States.

In 1963 it became clear that the nation's supply of physicians was inadequate to meet its health care needs. The principal evidence was shortages in nonurban areas and in primary care. Not only was it difficult to find a physician who made house calls, but in more and more communities it was difficult to find a physician. Congress, over the continuing objections of the AMA, passed the Health Professions Educational Assistance Act to provide matching grants for the construction, expansion, and renovation of health professionals schools, and federal loans for students in medicine, osteopathy, and dentistry. Again Congress began modestly with an initial authorization of only $30 million in fiscal year 1964. Within a decade Congress had approved five additional pieces of health manpower legislation to support medical and other health professional schools and raise total annual appropriations to well over $1.5 billion. Included in this legislation were capitation grants paid to medical schools for each medical student enrolled, which proved an extremely strong incentive for the schools to expand enrollment. The excess supply of physicians in the 1980s and'90s resulted in large part from these capitation grants.

Of course, direct congressional support for biomedical research waned during the mid-1960s as the new political fad moved to human resource support for improvement in and better access to health care delivery, and especially for the newly (1969) created family physician specialty. The result of 20 years of increased federal support of health manpower was to expand the nation's educational capacity for producing physicians, dentists, nurses, and other allied health care personnel. The number of students in medical school more than doubled between 1965 and 1980. Dental school enrollment increased fivefold, and nursing school enrollment increased by more than 75 percent. By 1980 this increased educational capacity had produced a substantially higher ratio of physicians, dentists, and nurses to population (39.9, 29.4, and 75.5 percent higher, respectively). The only elusive goal was to increase the relative percent of physicians practicing primary rather than specialty care, but the specialists were moving into less urban areas, which alleviated some of the physician shortages in these communities.

Except for its support of hospital and clinic facilities, the federal government's track record for benevolence programs was rather checkered. The lack of clear program objectives, a way of monitoring results, and a method for fine-tuning program expenditures to meet modified objectives was no doubt the primary failing of the federal government. The federal dollars were being invested in the principal resources of the nation's health care delivery system—manpower, facilities, and technology. The rapid rate of investment, coupled with violent swings in the type of resource support, proved to be very destabilizing to the health care industry. Such wild fluctuations of investment would disrupt any private market. The roller-coaster effect of federal government involvement would be equally overwhelming and destabilizing when it finally chose to enter the health care market as a purchaser of care for the aged and poor.

Postwar Hospital Development

Almost by default the hospital after World War II became the only mainstream institution in medical practice that served an integrating role in the health care industry. During the postwar period, "the

TABLE 3.3   Changing Role of the Hospital in the Health Care Sector For
Selected Years between 1929–1960

Year	Hosp. Expen. as % Health Care Expend.*	Gen Hosp Adm per 1,000**	Gen Hosp PD per 1,000***
1929	18.1%	56.3	701
1940	25.1	74.3	900
1950	30.7	110.5	898
1960	32.9	128.9	978

Sources: Expenditure data U.S. Department of Health, Education, and Welfare [1973],
and hospital utilization data from E. L. Corwin [1946, 84-90] and various issues of
American Hospital Association, *Hospitals*, August 1, Part 2.

   *Hospital Expenditures as a Percentage of Health Care Expenditures
  **General Hospital Admissions per 1,000 (population)
 ***General Hospital Patient Days per 1,000 (population)

hospital . . . [became] . . . an essential resource for medical practice
in America" [Freymann 1974, 68]. The relative importance of the hospital in the health care industry is reflected by the increasing share of
expenditures for hospital care out of total health care expenditures in
the United States. Table 3.3 suggests that the hospital sector experienced the largest relative growth over other types of health care expenditures in the 1930s and 1940s. Its relative share of the health care dollar
rose from 18 percent in 1929 to 25 percent in 1940, thus surpassing
expenditures for physicians as the leading component of health care
spending and to nearly one-third of all spending in 1960.

     The data on general hospital utilization per capita suggest that
two kinds of growth occurred in the 1930s and 1940s. In the '30s the
primary cause of greater spending on hospital care was increased
utilization of the hospital, which rose from just 700 days of care per
1,000 people to 900 days of care. The increase in the number of persons
admitted to the hospital in the 1930s was even greater than the per
capita days of care would suggest because the number of admissions
per capita was rising even more rapidly as the average length of stay
per admission was falling from about 15 days to less than 13 in 1940.

     The average length of stay continued to fall in the 1940s and
1950s, with the exception of the wartime period. A significant source
of increased inpatient hospital utilization resulted from the rising birth
rate after World War II and the increased use of the hospital for

newborn deliveries. Corwin [1946, 92] reports that only about 40 percent of all births took place in the hospital in 1935. According to the AHA hospital births rose to over 75 percent in 1950 and to more than 90 percent in 1960. During this period the rising number of maternity admissions, with their short stay, contributed substantially to the falling average length of stay for the whole hospital.

The principal cause of increased hospital expenditures to total health care expenditures in the 1940s was twofold: a continued increase in the number of persons admitted to hospitals and the hospital's growing role as the integrator of health care services. As noted earlier, nursing services in the 1940s moved into the hospital from its independent practice status. Thus consumer expenditures for nursing service became a part of hospital services in calculating national health expenditures. The addition of nursing service to the hospital virtually doubled hospital salary expenses—the annual rate of short-term general hospital expenses exceeded 20 percent in the three years, 1946–1948, immediately after the war. The hospital's level of health care expenditures also rose as a result of the increased dispensing of drugs to its patients. In 1956, hospitals dispensed almost one-quarter of all prescription pharmaceutical sales [The Somers 1961, 94–95].

In addition to assuming activities that had been carried out by other sectors of the health care industry, hospitals grew by inaugurating a host of new diagnostic procedures and more invasive surgical and other therapies. A prime example of the more invasive surgical procedures was Blalock's first "blue baby" operation at Johns Hopkins Hospital in 1944. A decade later open-heart surgery employing the heart-lung pump was available, and the first kidney transplant was made at the Peter Bent Brigham Hospital in Boston. Although surgery was expanding anatomically and in complexity—more than one-half of the nation's short-term general hospitals had postoperative recovery rooms—hospitals were becoming less dependent on surgeons for inpatient admissions. In the early 1930s surgical admissions had represented nearly 75 percent of all hospital admissions. By the late 1950s only 60 percent of hospital admissions had surgery, a figure that would drop to 50 percent of the admissions in another decade [The Somers 1961, 65].

Laboratory and radiological diagnostic procedures were becoming more important to the hospital's product line. The number of lab tests per admission rose from an average of 4 in 1946 to 14 in 1958

[The Somer 1961, 69]. Hospitals were also replacing the physician's house calls through their emergency rooms, especially on weekends and in the evening.

Hospitals not only redesigned their services and facilities to meet the changing practice patterns of the postwar physician specialist, they also altered the way their services were provided in order to attract more physicians to the community. House staff available to hospitals through the expanded number of residency programs was perhaps the best means of increasing a given hospital's relative attractiveness for medical staff appointments. Meeting specialty board standards for residencies enhanced the hospital's prestige in the medical community, and filling the approved residencies with young specialty physicians provided 24-hour on-call service for the medical staff's private patients.

The competitive advantage of the graduate teaching hospital over rival community hospitals was significant both in terms of prestige and the economic advantages the residents brought to the hospital's private medical staff. Although hospitals without approved residency programs were at a competitive disadvantage, the growing role of allied health professions in the delivery of health and medical care offered these hospitals an alternative means of competing for medical staff. The practice of a more technical form of medicine required more allied support personnel in medical practice, and these support personnel were also becoming more specialized. The ratio of health care workers to physicians and dentists rose from 4.1 in 1930 [Falk et al 1928, 519–520] to 4.8 in 1955 [The Somers 1961, 539].

Hospitals became the principal employers of the allied health personnel who provided support services to physicians. In 1930 hospitals had employed less than one-third of all health workers, but by 1955 almost two-thirds of all health workers were employed by the nation's hospitals. Although some of this increase simply represented a change in the employment status of nurses, an important part of the increase in hospital employment was the growing numbers of lab, x-ray, and other technicians needed to render postwar institutional health care.

The increasing technical-integrative role of the hospital during the postwar period was also reflected in the type of capital equipment and facilities invested in hospitals. In the 20 years from 1928 to 1948, the assets that short-term general hospitals had invested per bed increased only about 17 percent in real terms. However, in the 12 years from 1948 to 1960 the real investment per bed increased by more than 50 percent. The acute general hospital was becoming a much more intensive technological resource for community health care.

The substantially larger capital requirements for hospital operations coupled with the severe capital shortage for hospital investment during the Great Depression produced a huge backlog of capital needs, which some areas of the private sector would have had difficulty in meeting. Obsolete plant facilities at the end of World War II that constituted a public hazard represented about one-sixth of all available hospital beds, and the total stock of beds was estimated to provide less than two-thirds of the total beds needed [The Laves 1974, 25]. The perceived shortage in beds was further exacerbated by a maldistribution of hospital facilities that caused rural areas to experience much more acute shortages than urban areas.

The Hill-Burton program was politically popular, and a number of poorer rural communities, especially, were able to construct new hospitals under its aegis, and other communities may have replaced their older facilities more rapidly. "Between 1949 and 1962, about 30 percent of all hospital construction projects were assisted . . . [or] . . . about 10 percent of the annual cost of all hospital construction over this period was paid directly by the federal government under the Hill-Burton program" [The Laves 1974, 16]. Nevertheless, the financial viability of the older hospitals was probably sufficient to have financed most of these capital expenditures without federal assistance.

Although patient revenues throughout the period were less than total operating expenses, on average total revenues exceeded expenses by about 3 percent. In addition, the hospitals entered the decade of the 1960s with virtually no long-term debt [Foster 1976]. The widespread coverage of hospital insurance for the employed population had, indeed, provided a secure foundation to the financing of acute hospital care for most American communities. Hill-Burton grants and community philanthropy added sufficiently to this base to allow the hospitals the luxury of avoiding long-term debt commitments.

The coalescing of one-third of the nation's health care expenditures under the fiscally strong umbrella of the hospitals, coupled with the significant growth of professional hospital administrators as their managers, might suggest that the hospitals had realized their earlier promise to become the organizational focus and entrepreneur for the nation's health care system. However, the hospital remained instead the site for centralizing acute health care services and the community's highly technical and specialized human resources. It was still basically the physician's workshop with little managerial and virtually no entrepreneurial control over the medical activities conducted in the institution.

The Postwar Consumer

Although much of the increase in utilization of the short-term acute hospital occurred in the 1930s, the postwar period was marked by a pronounced change in the consumer's attitude toward the medical care system. The use of its technological resources in the treatment of illness, as exemplified earlier by the change in choice of hospital versus home deliveries that occurred in this period, also played a role. The number of doctor visits per capita more than doubled, and the percentage of persons seeing a doctor at least once a year increased from less than 50 percent in the late 1920s and early 1930s [Falk et al 1928, 64] to more than 64 percent in 1963 [Andersen et al 1968, 17].

Perhaps the most important single event in the consumer's perception of the benefit of health care therapies was the diffusion of the wonder drugs and their effectiveness in combatting infectious diseases. The dramatic effect of some surgical interventions, such as the "blue baby" operation, further enhanced the physician's image during the postwar years. However, access to the miracles of modern medicine was not uniformly distributed across American society. The wealthier and better educated were much more likely to seek medical assistance for illness, but there was mounting evidence that the lower-income groups would seek care if the rising financial barriers to care were removed [The Somers 1961, 155].

Health insurance coverage in 1965 extended to nearly 72 percent of the population for hospitalization and more than 45 percent for medical/surgical benefits. The consumer's out-of-pocket costs for personal health care, as Table 3.4 reports, were approaching one half of total health care expenditures. However, the effect of health insurance varied significantly by the kind of insurance and the kind of health care expenditure. Consumers' out-of-pocket hospital expenses were only about 20 percent of total hospital expenses, but slightly more than 60 percent of physician expenditures. In 1960 consumers spent only $1.9 billion for hospital care with a total cost to society of $9.3 billion. On the other hand, they spent $3.3 billion in out-of-pocket

TABLE 3.4   Sources of Financing Personal Health Care for Selected Years between 1940–1965

Year	Consumer	Private Insurance	Government	Total Exp.*	Annual % Chg.
1940	82.0%	—	15.3%	$ 3.4	
1950	68.3	8.5%	20.2%	10.4	11.8%
1955	59.0	15.5	22.8	15.2	7.9
1960	55.3	20.7	21.8	22.7	8.4
1965	52.5	24.7	20.8	33.5	8.1

Source: U.S. Department of Health, Education, and Welfare, 1972.

*Total Expenditures in billions of dollars

payments for physician care, typically rendered in the hospital, that only cost $5.3 billion in total. The health insurance benefits structure was encouraging both consumers and physicians to utilize the most expensive form of care in order to qualify for insurance coverage.

The consumer, by the structure of health insurance, was being directed toward the hospital and the practitioners of scientific medicine who were overrepresented on hospital medical staffs. The GPs and internists, who practiced primarily on an outpatient or ambulatory basis, received little in the way of health insurance payments. Therefore, if the consumer chose care out of the hospital, it could cost the consumer more even though it cost much less in total than the cost of that same treatment provided in the hospital.

ESTABLISHING THE LAUNCHING PAD FOR EXPLOSIVE GROWTH: A SUMMARY OF THE FIRST GROWTH PHASE

By most industries' standards the health care industry's growth in the 25 years after 1940 was phenomenal. It would have been almost impossible to imagine in 1965 that this period had simply been a prelude to a much larger growth phase that would eventually endanger the fiscal integrity of most middle class Americans and even the budget of the mighty federal government. The only hint that such explosive growth was in store for the health care industry was the industry's failure to change its organizational structure during the 20 postwar years. The industry was structured almost exactly as it had been at the end of the 1920s with physicians working solo on a piece-

TABLE 3.5 Personal Health Care Expenditures for Hospitals, Physicians, and Drugs in Selected Years between 1940–1965

Year	Personal Health Expenditures		Hospital Expenditures		Physician Expenditures		Drug Expenditures	
	Billions	% Chg*	Billions	% Chg*	Billions	% Chg*	Billions	% Chg*
1940	$ 3.4		$ 1.0		$ .9		$ .6	
1950	10.4	12.2	3.7	14.0	2.7	11.6	1.6	10.3
1955	15.2	7.9	5.7	9.0	3.6	6.2	2.3	7.0
1960	22.7	8.4	8.5	8.4	5.6	9.0	3.6	9.5
1965	33.5	8.1%	13.2	9.1%	8.4	8.5%	4.6	5.3%

Source: U.S. Department of Health, Education, and Welfare [1976] for the 1950 to 1965 years and Levit et al [1985] for 1970. *The percentage change for each five-year period has been coverted to an average annual rate of increase for the four expenditure categories.

work basis and freely utilizing the hospital as their principal workshop for major medical interventions.

Between 1940 to 1965 was a period of consolidating support for scientific medicine among consumers, insurance carriers, employers, and agencies of government. Each of these groups, whether aware or not, enthusiastically bought into the previous agreements between doctors and hospitals that had tempered competition in the health care industry. The key was, of course, freedom-of-choice health insurance in which all the parties cooperated, even to the extent of employers' assuming the risk-bearing function. Hospitals and the doctors who practice in them had achieved a general buy-in to their preferred method of organization, gained a relative riskless financing mechanism, and more federal dollars than could be spent wisely.

In spite of these expansionary conditions, the rate of increase for personal health care expenditures, except for the decade of the 40s with its wartime dislocations, was held to approximately 8 percent, as indicated in Table 3.5. Because of the labor intensity of health care services and the need to match wages based on productivity increases in a manufacturing dominated economy and because of the substantial improvement in the value of health services, this pace of unit cost increase and growth in the quantity of services provided was not unreasonable [Baumol 1993]. Further, U.S. health care spending in 1965 was generally consistent with the level of spending in other developed nations.

If there were any inconsistencies, it was the allocation of resources within the health care industry, not the total amount of resources being spent on health care. Scientific medicine, with its emphasis on specialization, technology, and the hospital, was winning all the competitive battles without any active campaign.

Meanwhile the AMA continued to campaign against voluntary health insurance benefits covering its general practitioner constituency and federal support for graduate medical education. Its efforts were leading the GPs and other primary care physicians into an untenable position in the health care marketplace, which would have serious implications for the future of the health care industry and the national budget during the remainder of the 20th century.

4

The Exploding Market for Health Services, 1966–1979

The health care industry's second growth phase occurred in two quite different stages. The first was a continuation, but at an accelerated pace, of the postwar pattern. That is, there was simply a higher rate of expansion for the scientific medicine/hospital model of health care as a result the federal government's huge incremental investment in health care through the 1965 passage of the Medicare entitlement for the aged and the Medicaid welfare program for the poor. Because the universal benefits for the aged emulated all the past accommodations in the private health insurance market—low or first-dollar coverage without adequate provider cost controls or incentives for efficient health care delivery—it gave the coup de grace to effective competition in the health care marketplace. These federal programs have ratchet-like benefits for the aged that can only expand and never contract. They have spread the past private market accommodations that stifled competition across the entire health care market, created frictionless inflationary market conditions, and made effective reform of the health care market extremely difficult.

This chapter first describes how the legislative design of the Medicare-Medicaid programs produced a great leap upward in the rate of health care inflation. The political popularity of employer-sponsored health insurance model when applied to the poor and the aged had two conflicting results—a great potential for inflationary, demand-driven increases in health care services and a significant improvement in the health status of older and poorer Americans. The second section of the chapter traces the disparate responses of government and providers to the huge increase in the demand for health care services. And finally, the third section of the chapter outlines the structural changes in the health care market that grew out of these new federal programs.

EXPANSION OF HEALTH CARE DEMAND

The Legislative History of Medicare

Federal enactment of health insurance for the aged was foreordained by the success of private health insurance for employee groups and the incompatibility of experience rating that was used in pricing that insurance for older, retired employees, whose average health care costs were twice as high as for the under 65-year olds. When it became apparent that a federal universal health insurance program could not be approved, attention turned to providing health insurance for the aged. Public health insurance for the aged was first introduced in Congress in 1956 and became a major campaign issue in both the 1960 and 1964 presidential elections. Thus, civil servants in the Social Security Administration and the Department of Health, Education, and Welfare had been planning Medicare for many years before its passage.

This long and difficult legislative history was due primarily to the AMA's zealous opposition. Finally after Lyndon Johnson's landslide victory in 1964, Congressman Wilbur Mills of Arkansas, the astute chairman of the House Ways and Means Committee, found the magic combination of program benefits, financing, and administrative structure to assure its overwhelming approval.[8] Mills combined hospital insurance coverage financed through the social security system with voluntary medical insurance financed by subscriber premiums and general tax revenues to provide those 65 and over with comprehensive health insurance (Medicare Part A for hospital benefits and Part B for medical benefits). He then folded in an upgraded federal-state matching program to provide health insurance benefits to the medically indigent (Medicaid) [Richard Harris 1966 and Peter A. Corning 1969]. Medicaid replaced the Kerr-Mills matching program that had been enacted in 1960 but not completely implemented by all the states.

Congress only had to choose between accommodating the interests of physicians or hospitals on a single issue. Once Mills had divided Medicare into separate programs—a compulsory hospital and a voluntary medical program—a determination had to be made as to whether hospital-based physicians, e.g., pathologists and radiologists, would be placed in Part A and Part B. Mills chose to keep all physician benefits in Part B, and he defeated in the conference committee a Senate proposal (the Douglas amendment) to make all hospital services Part A benefits. This decision created the first public crack in the pre-1920 hospital-medical staff alliance, but the broad ambulatory insurance coverage provided in Part B would eventually place an even greater strain on the traditional doctor-hospital relationship. Only one other major controversy arose during the administrative implementation of the program, and that concerned hospital reimbursement.[9]

On July 1, 1966, M-day as the Johnson Administration labeled it, Medicare began very smoothly, including the racial integration of all the nation's health facilities without rancor or incident, and Medicaid began six months later. Congress,[10] and Mills, had crafted an extremely popular program for aged beneficiaries and their offspring, who no longer were contingently liable for their parents' medical bills. At the time many veterans of the national health insurance campaign believed that the younger citizens' observation of the seniors' financial bliss would lead to the demand for universal coverage within a short time.

The forecast of renewed demand for universal coverage was correct as to timing, but wholly incorrect as to why. The primary motive in the late '60s and early '70s for seeking universal health insurance coverage was the perceived failings, not the successes, of Medicare and Medicaid programs. The principal failing and earliest observable effect of the new programs was the immediate and substantial increase in health care and, especially, hospital costs. The lack of cost containment was rooted in the original program design, not in the programs' benevolent implementation. Although SSA officials worked very closely and cooperatively with trade association representatives of doctors and hospitals in the development of the Medicare program's administrative regulations, the program latitudes proposed at that time were minor in comparison to the inflationary concessions made by Congress in drafting the original legislation. Hospitals were to be paid on a full-cost recovery basis, and doctors were to be paid on a "usual and customary" fee basis. Blue Cross/Blue Shield plans and private health insurance companies won the role of administrative intermediaries between SSA and the providers to give a government program the appearance and feel of the traditional private sector operations, and the Medicare insurance benefits were patterned after the Blues' first-dollar service benefit approach. Emulation of what had worked in the private sector had been Congress' credo in drafting the legislation to not only reach accommodation with health care providers, but to make it as much like what consumers had experienced from their previous employer-financed health insurance programs.

The use of the private health insurance prototype for constructing the first public health insurance in the United States failed to recognize that:

> For all practical purposes there were no controls on the providers. Hospitals were paid cost or charges, whichever was lower; physicians were paid their usual and customary fees. The economy was expansive enough in the forties, at least for the burgeoning voluntary health insurance plans, that hard bargaining with providers was neither necessary nor practical. The funding sources [primarily, employers] went along [Anderson 1985, 263].

Implementing a huge new federal health insurance program without effective provider cost controls eliminated virtually all remaining cost restraints in the U.S. health care system. The first or low dollar coverage, especially of Blue Cross and Blue Shield plans, had already insulated the consumer from cost considerations in selecting health care providers and treatment regimens. A health care delivery and financing system that protected both affluent Americans and health care providers from cost concerns, coupled with an aged constituency that resisted benefit reductions or increased cost sharing, left, as we shall see, few alternatives for government to contain health care costs.

The Medicare Cost Explosion

In the five years before the implementation of Medicare and Medicaid, the rate of growth in personal health care expenditures had slowed somewhat to just over 8 percent per year. From 1965 to 1970 it jumped to 14.4 percent. Although physician and drug expenditures also rose by double-digit annual rates (11.2 and 11.5 percent, respectively), the average annual increase in expenditures for hospital care from 1965 to 1970 was the largest rate of increase both in absolute terms, 16.3 percent, and in rate of increase over the pre-Medicare rate of growth, more than 85 percent higher than the 1950 to 1965 annual rate of 8.8 percent.

Table 4.1 provides data on the utilization of the nonfederal short-term general hospital from 1950–1975 as well as the average expense per admission for five-year intervals.

TABLE 4.1   Hospital Utilization and Expenses For Selected Years between 1950–1975

Year	Adm per 1,000*	P.D. per 1,000**	Millions of Admissions	Annual % Change	Expense per Adm	Annual % Change
1950	110.5	898	16.663	—	$ 127	—
1955	117.2	909	19.100	2.8%	180	7.4%
1960	128.7	978	22.970	3.7	245	6.3
1965	138.2	1,071	26.463	2.9	316*	7.1**
1970	145.1	1,194	29.252	2.2	605*	13.8*
1975	158.6	1,225	33.519	2.8	1,025*	11.1*

Source: American Hospital Association, *AHA Hospital Statistics*, 1991–1992 edition, for nonfederal short-term general hospitals. *Calculated for adjusted admissions, which takes into account outpatient operating expenses. **Calculated without taking outpatient operating expenses into account.

*Admissions per 1,000 (population)
**Patient Days per 1,000 (population)

The generally-accepted explanation for the higher rate of hospital expenditure increases after World War II was the higher rate of increased demand for hospital services than for other goods and services in the economy. Martin Feldstein [1971], for example, has concluded:

> Increasing demand has been identified as the primary reason for the unusually rapid rate of cost increase. Rising income and more comprehensive insurance coverage, both private and public, have increased patients' willingness to pay for more and better hospital care. The result has been a small rise in per capita days [from 898 per 1,000 population in 1950 to 1,225 in 1975 or about 1.25 percent annual rate of growth in per capita hospital days over the 25 year period] and a substantial increase in the cost per day [or stay] of hospital care. Higher demand has induced a

change in the technology of hospital care to a better but more expensive product.

By technology change Feldstein meant that the character of hospital services has changed as reflected in an increasing number and kind of inputs used to produce those services. Hospitals were adding services, such as intensive care beds, more sophisticated imaging equipment, nuclear therapy, and renal dialysis facilities, that required more inputs per patient day or stay and thus raised hospital unit and total costs at a rate higher than growth in the rest of the economy. Feldstein and Taylor [1977, 20] found that 75 percent of the unit cost increases in this period stemmed from "the growing number of employees and the increasing volumes of equipment and supplies rather than the rise in the price of these inputs."

Paradoxically, hospitals in more competitive markets were under greater pressure to "provide higher levels of both patient- and physician-oriented services than hospitals whose access to patients is less threatened" [Robinson and Luft 1987, 3241]. That is, competition in the hospital marketplace worked perversely to increase costs rather than to minimize cost as expected in competitive markets. This perverse behavior is a result of the consumers (patients) being insulated from cost considerations due to health insurance and hospitals in multihospital markets competing for the consumer's agents (physicians) by providing services that are attractive in recruiting physicians to their medical staffs.[11]

The effect of the Medicaid and, especially, the Medicare program was to greatly expand demand for hospital services and to accelerate the rate of growth in hospital expenditure and the number and sophistication of hospital services beyond the levels that had been experienced from 1950 to 1965 when more gradual increases in private insurance coverage and family income occurred. The two groups covered by the new federal programs, the poor and the aged, were "historically heavy utilizers of hospital service. However, with the introduction of Medicare and Medicaid, utilization increased markedly; for example, the number of days of hospital care per 1,000 aged persons rose 24.8 percent between 1965 and 1967. This tremendous increase in the demand for hospital care [and further reductions in price or cost sensitivity] produced the largest rate of increase in hospital expenditures since the immediate post-World War II period" [Drake and Raske 1974].

The Medicare-Medicaid Health Dividend

Adding the poor and the aged to the U.S. hospital-based health insurance system proved to be extremely expensive. It also produced substantial budget overruns for the programs and ushered in a new era in the debate over national health insurance. However, often overlooked in the review of the programs because of their high cost and delays in reporting is their effect on the health of the American people. Table 4.2 shows that there had been no significant improvement in the nation's age-adjusted mortality rates since 1955 when the effect of antibiotics on infectious diseases had been fully absorbed. During the decade after the implementation of the Medicare and Medicaid programs the United States experienced a greater increase in relative life expectancy for 80-year-olds than other comparable developed nations; a greater increase in 60-year-olds life expectancy than any other developed country except Japan; and a substantial (34.8 percent) reduction in infant mortality, as did France, Japan, and Sweden. In comparison to our own health indicators, these 10 years produced "more than one-third of the total increased longevity achieved

TABLE 4.2   U.S. Mortality Rates for Selected Years between 1940–80

Year	Age-adjusted Death Rate per 1,000	Percentage Decrease
1940	10.8	—
1945	9.5	12.0%
1950	8.4	11.6
1955	7.7	8.3
1960	7.6	1.3
1965	7.4	2.6
1970	7.1	4.1
1975	6.7	9.9
1980	5.9	11.9

Source: U.S. Department of Health, Education, and Welfare [1977, 14] and U.S. Department of Commerce [1992].

by a 65-year-old in the first 75 years of this century," and the rate of decrease in infant mortality during these 10 years was more than twice the rate that had been accomplished in the 15 years from 1950 to 1965, with a disproportionate improvement for nonwhite infants, which was four times as great as their improvement in the preceding 15 years [Drake 1978, 64–65].

The key to the improvement in health from these two programs was that poorer Americans benefited the most. Medicaid was directed by statute to lower-income groups, but it was also lower-income aged persons who increased their hospital and doctor utilization. Although the total number of physician visits, 6.6 per year, by persons 65 and older did not change between 1965 and 1975, "the number of physician contacts per year per person increased for the elderly poor and decreased for the nonpoor . . . thus differences in the physician utilization by the poor and nonpoor elderly have been narrowed or elminated" [Kovar 1977, 14].

On the other hand, hospital utilization over the first decade increased substantially. There was a 36 percent increase in per capita aged admissions and a 21 percent increase in aged patient days from 1965 to 1975, but the admission rate for the poor aged increased by 47 percent and the nonpoor elderly rate only increased 18 percent over the 11 years beginning in 1964. The greater utilization of hospital services may not only have contributed to longer expected life for the poor aged, but also to their quality of life as illustrated by a doubling in the rate of cataract surgery for the aged and a tripling in the rate of arthroplasty. In 1975 more than two-thirds of the noninstitutionalized elderly (95 percent) rated their health as good or excellent, and only 9 percent rated it poor. The poorer elderly did, however, rate their health status slightly less favorably across the board [Kovar 1977].

SEARCHING FOR THE BRAKES

Whether or not the benefits of these programs required a double-digit rate of increases in health care costs is arguable. However, the broad kind of health improvements that took place were not known during the initial stages of the cost containment debate that was launched in the late '60s and throughout the decade of the 1970s. Medicare was so popular that Congress has never considered reducing its program benefits. Medicaid, however, has experienced many cutbacks. Both federal and state governments have periodically raised entitlement qualifications, lowered state program requirements, and/or introduced limitations on some Medicaid benefits despite the evidence that making health care available to the poor has by far the bigger payoff in terms of improved health.[12] Except for tinkering with the Medicaid benefits, the principal thrust of congressional cost containment efforts was directed at health care providers and a new strategy of shifting government program costs to the private sector, mainly to the policy holders of private health insurance.

Changing Role of Government

The 1968 election of President Richard Nixon brought to an abrupt end the expansionist health policies of the Great Society. After less than three months in office, the new administration stunned hospitals when Robert Finch, Secretary of Health, Education, and Welfare, announced the elimination of the plus factor from the Medicare cost reimbursement formula, effective July 1, 1969. Although the ensuing dispute was settled later in the year, it dramatized the different attitudes about government spending between the Nixon and Johnson Administrations. Johnson had thought of Medicare as part of his "youthful dream of improving life for more people and in more ways than any other political leader, including FDR" [Leuchtenbury 1983, p. 142]. Nixon saw it as a drain on the federal treasury that needed to be plugged. However, the new government effort to contain health care costs was interpreted narrowly, much as a private market oligopsonist (few major purchasers of a product) would seek to minimize its share of total hospital costs, and not as a government regulator with broad public responsibility for reducing the overall cost of the nation's health care.

In the case of hospital costs, for example, the federal government first focused on its own program costs, not on an overall strategy to reduce society's health care costs. "Through imaginative and selective changes in the accounting and apportionment techniques, HEW was able to reduce the federal government's share of total hospital costs [from] . . . 92 percent of a hospital's average per diem cost in 1966 to 80 percent in 1977" [Drake 1980]. The federal government's efforts to minimize its programs' share of health care costs led hospitals to increase the charges to private health insurance programs and the increasingly smaller group of self-pay patients in order to recover their costs.

This practice, known as "cost shifting," in turn led a rising number of state governments to consider and implement broader regulations to reduce the rate of overall increase in hospital costs, first through areawide planning controls on capital investments in facilities and equipment and then on the prices of hospital services. New York was the first state to impose investment controls in 1964, even before the Medicare cost explosion. Nineteen other states followed in the late '60s and early '70s.

Although rate regulation followed investment or planning controls, in varying degrees rates were regulated by 1976 "for over one-fourth of the nation's hospitals, located in 28 states" [American Hospital Association, 1977, 174]. Connecticut, Maryland, Massachusetts, New Jersey, New York, and Washington imposed the earliest and most comprehensive rate regulation programs. Because rate regulation had the potential for both reducing the rate of price increases and achieving greater equity or parity among all purchaser groups, the Health Insurance Association of America, the trade association for the commercial health insurance companies, became the leading spokesman for public utility type regulation of the hospital industry. However, periodically during the '70s, the American Hospital Association, the largest and predominant hospital trade association, also supported public-utility type regulation of hospitals [Lovinger 1985]. Because a secondary effect of cost shifting had inflated the differential or discount that advantaged Blue Cross plans in their competition with the commercial carriers, it was very much in the interests of HIAA's members to pursue public utility-type rate regulation at the state level.

While many states were developing regulatory programs to control hospital capital investments and regulate rates for private purchasers of hospital care, President Nixon declared a health care cost crisis in July 1969. The Congress, starting in February 1970 with a report on Medicare and Medicaid by the staff of the Senate Finance Committee, began hearings on how it could bring federal program costs under control. The report laid out an array of problems, starting with a need to double the rate of Medicare payroll taxes because of hospital and nursing home cost overruns. It took the Congress nearly three years before legislative remedies could be agreed upon, and the 1972 Amendments to the Social Security Act were passed in October of that year. In its introduction Finance Committee staff concluded that "The key to making the present system workable and acceptable is the physician and his medical society . . . . In the absence of such constructive effort, we fear that virtually insurmountable pressures will develop for alternative control procedures which may be arbitrary, rigid and insensitive to the legitimate needs of both the patient and his physician" [U.S. Senate Finance Committee 1970].

As Congress proceeded to develop a regulatory program for federal programs and consider national health insurance proposals, the Administration developed a private market initiative through the proposed Health Maintenance Organizations (HMOs) Act[13] to control health care costs. This bill was initially approved in 1974, but it actually slowed HMO formation due to the rigid federal approval standards. An amendment to the act in 1978 gave some flexibility, and the appropriations for subsidizing the development of HMOs were also helpful in overcoming the dampening effect of the original legislation [Falkson 1980].

During the remainder of 1970 and through 1971, all these avenues—adding regulatory controls to the federal programs, the new HMO strategy for controlling costs through the marketplace, and various national health insurance proposals for both controlling costs and providing universal access to health care—were explored. However, on August 15, 1971, President Nixon, who had launched the HMO strategy in a health message to Congress in February, astonished the country by imposing a wage-price freeze on the economy. In 1970 the Democratic Congress had given the the president authority to impose wage and price controls to combat rising levels of inflation. Congress had intended to embarrass the president about inflation in the 1972 elections. No one had expected a Republican president to impose these controls, which had always been anathema to free market Republicans. Nixon continued the program until April 30, 1974, when the presidential authority for wage and price regulation was allowed to expire and he was deeply engrossed in his handling of the Watergate scandal.

Only the health care industry was subjected to all four phases of the Economic Stablization Program (ESP) over the full 990 days of its duration. Although he was ideologically opposed, President Nixon imposed a full-scale, comprehensive regulatory program on all the nation's health care providers for nearly three years. Ironically, this regulatory initiative had only a negligible effect on restraining the inflationary spiral of health care costs.

The remainder of the 1970s, with the exception of the original HMO Act of 1974 and its amendment in 1978, was spent either with legislative bodies debating additional regulatory controls for hospitals or with the executive branches of federal and state governments implementing new regulatory programs. In October 1972, Congress finally approved omnibus regulatory controls after two and one-half years of debate. The Social Security Amendments of 1972 was primarily a cost containment proposal, but it also contained two major new health entitlements—a Medicare entitlement for persons eligible for federal disability coverage and a new program entitlement for persons suffering from end-stage renal disease (untreatable kidney failure). The latter program would have important implications for subsequent hospital-physician relations.

The Social Security Amendments included the following cost controls: limitations on routine inpatient service costs, physician payments in teaching hospitals, and the lower of cost or charges for hospitals services; a new organization, the Professional Standards Review Organization (PSRO), to substitute external review of hospital utilization for the hospital's own peer review committees; and a linkage to areawide planning agencies to deny capital payments for projects that had been disapproved by planning agencies. The latter control device was extended through the federalization of health planning in the United States by the National Health Planning and Resources Development Act of 1974, which was signed into law by President Gerald Ford in January 1975. Federal planning sought to reduce the rate of investment in health facilities and was a bonanza for lawyers and accountants who assisted hospitals through the maze of regulatory review on a consulting basis.

The election of Jimmy Carter in 1976 only intensified the regulatory debate as Carter made his proposed Hospital Cost Containment Act the highest health legislative priority. With HEW Secretary Joseph A. Califano, Jr. leading the charge, the debate over these controls reached a fever pitch. Animosity between the Carter White House and the private health sector became fierce by the time the House of Representatives rejected Carter's proposal. Instead of enacting mandatory controls, the House accepted a voluntary program as a substitute on November 15, 1979. A watershed in the political fortunes of hospitals was reached that day.

Multihospital Systems

While government reacted to the initial Medicare cost bulge by considering and enacting various cost control regulations, the private market responded to the increased demand for institutional health care by increased investment in institutional health care facilities. Between 1965 and 1970 total assets of nonfederal short-term general and other special hospitals increased by 63 percent, and beds increased by 14.4 percent. During the next five years there was an even higher rate of growth in total assets, 77.2 percent, and only slightly smaller growth in beds, 11.7 percent. The rapid expansion continued through the remainder of the 1970s in spite of ESP and the rising number of state and federal investment controls, but at diminished rates of increase. The total supply of short-term general hospital beds did not stop growing until 1983 when the number of beds peaked at just over one million.

The need for capital to finance this expansion in community hospitals and nursing home facilities led to the first major change in hospital ownership since the Great Depression of the 1930s—the revival of the for-profit hospital. At this stage, however, instead of small sole proprietorships, investor-owned multihospital systems were developed. These systems had the advantage of raising equity capital through the sale of stock on the national exchanges and then leveraging that equity capital through the issuance of long-term debt instruments.

Proprietary or for-profit hospitals, as they were called prior to Medicare, together with for-profit nursing homes lobbied Congress in 1966 to amend the hospital reimbursement provisions by adding a rate of return on equity (equal to 1.5 times the rate of earnings that the federal government received on the Medicare trust fund) as part of their allowable patient care costs in place of one-quarter of the 2 percent allowance in lieu of specific costs; i.e., they continued to receive a 1.5 percent allowance until it was eliminated in 1969.

Because reimbursement of all reasonable costs plus a 1.5 percent allowance was assured together with the rate of return on investment, investors had a sure thing. Here was a virtually riskless investment alternative that could be purchased through the issuance of highly levered stock; i.e., stock that represented only a small portion of the total investment with the remainder financed through debt capital, and all reasonable interest charges were included in the reimbursement formula.

By 1968 and 1969 all the large multihospital chains had been formed. In the make-believe market of reasonable cost reimbursement, there wasn't even much pressure on how much was paid for the facilities. In fact, during the early years of the program, profits could be made by different chains buying each other out, which simply raised reasonable costs and owners' equity. Because of the fundamental soundness of the financial plan, chain company stocks became the darlings of the stock market, and substantial appreciation was realized.

To maintain the appreciated stock values, it became necessary for the chains to show increased earnings over time, and the simplest way to increase earnings was through growth in their hospital investment. However, during the '70s the available stock of proprietary hospitals suitable for investment was bought up by competing chains. The only remaining means of expansion was through the construction of new hospital facilities or the purchase of non-profit hospitals. The primary means for continued growth was the construction of new hospital facilities, especially in growing suburban communities in the Sun Belt and the purchase of or merger with other chains.

The entire inpatient hospital industry ceased growing in the 1980s. When growth would produce the necessary increased earnings per share to maintain or raise market values the larger companies simply spun off or sold their less profitable hospitals; raised funds through employee pension funds; or, in the case of sales, retired debt with the proceeds and continued to report higher per share earnings.

At this time the claims of superior management for investor-owned facilities over not-for-profit hospitals was really tested. Unfortunately for many of these systems, especially the smaller ones, it was also the time when Medicare financing of hospital services switched from the relatively easy reasonable cost reimbursement to the much tougher target of prospective payment. The Wall Street romance with most investor-owned multihospital systems ended when the chains could no longer continue to report higher per share earnings, and a number of the smaller companies went into bankruptcy.

The investor-owned phenomenon certainly had a significant influence on the development of the health care industry, but it did not
drastically change the ownership makeup of the hospital industry. In
1965, the small sole proprietorship hospitals constituted 14.9 percent
of the number of hospitals and 6.3 percent of the total nonfederal
short-term general and other special hospital beds in the United States.
In 1990, they owned 13.9 percent of the hospitals and 10.9 percent of
the beds. As a result of the for-profit system development, for-profit
hospitals were larger, doubling in average size from 47 beds in 1965
to 101 beds in 1990, which accounted for the 4.6 percent increase in
their share of beds. They were located in growth areas of the Sun Belt;
maintained higher quality standards, as evidenced by the increased
percentage that were accredited by the Joint Commission on Accreditation of Healthcare Organizations; and undoubtedly were much better
managed than in 1965.

Despite the improvement in the condition and location of the
for-profit hospitals, perhaps the more significant effect of the investor-
owned systems was on their not-for-profit rivals. Because of the great
publicity, especially in the business trade press, about the investor-
owned chains bringing better management to the hospital industry,
the not-for-profit hospital began to emulate their organizational style
and practices. In the 1970s not-for-profit hospitals began the biggest
merger and multihospital system movement that the hospital industry
had ever experienced.[14]

Some not-for-profit hospitals had for decades been nominally
part of multihospital chains through central ownership, primarily hospitals owned by religious orders. Most, however, operated as freestanding, community-based institutions until the advent of for- profit
chains. As the first effect of the system movement on not-for-profits,
these institutions began to explore the advantages of more centrally
directed management and financing as a means of enhancing the
system's mission and improving operations. Restructuring of these
systems frequently led to more centralized accounting and capital
financing, with increased efficiencies. It could be argued that the
reason for these changes was as much a response to the national
financing program of Medicare as it was an emulation of the for-
profits' behavior.

However, the growth of systems among freestanding not-for-
profit hospitals that followed in the 1970s and the subsequent formation of alliances, either a group of freestanding hospitals or a group
of hospital systems that combined through their purchase of shares

in a cooperative or corporation, was frequently in direct response to the increasing number of for-profit chain hospitals in local markets. The number of freestanding hospitals owned by not-for-profit systems nearly tripled from 410 hospitals in 1965 to 1,113 hospitals in 1979 [AHA 1981].

The not-for-profit systems differed from the for-profits in several respects. These systems were generally smaller, averaging 4.9 hospitals with 1,140 beds versus for-profit systems with an average of 23 hospitals and 2,954 beds. The individual not-for-profit hospitals were on average larger than the for-profit hospitals, 227 beds versus 128 beds. The not-for-profit systems were much more geographically concentrated and much less likely to extend beyond a single state. Their larger size tended to give the for-profit systems an advantage in capital financing, facility construction, and purchasing; but the greater geographic concentration gave the not-for-profits a better opportunity to organize and rationalize the delivery of health care in local markets. The alliances were formed as another vehicle to offset the purchasing advantage of the for-profit systems, and tax-exempt revenue bonds were used as the not-for-profits' principal capital financing mechanism.

Neither system did much to help the hospital industry to develop an integrated comprehensive health care delivery and financing organization. These systems were formed by horizontal mergers (merging like institutions across the industry) rather than vertical mergers (merging different parts of the production or marketing process, up or down). Toward the end of the '70s and the early '80s several systems tried to integrate medical services and/or consumer financing/marketing into their delivery organizations, but none of the larger systems or alliances was successful in vertically integrating the delivery and financing of health care. Thus, the multi-hospital systems only achieved marginal increases in asset financing, purchasing, or construction efficiencies. Multihospital systems did not further hospitals' goal of vertically integrating health care delivery systems.

Skyrocketing Costs and Rising Political Pressure

The continuing double-digit increase in hospital costs was directly reflected in the industry's heightened difficulties with Congress. In defeating the Carter cost cap proposal in late 1979, hospital representatives had argued that voluntary restraint, which had appeared to offer some relief in 1977 and 1978, would be sufficient to dampen the rate of increase in hospital costs. All the news after the House vote, however, indicated that the rate of increase in costs was rising, not falling. President Carter, even though he was in an all-out fight with Senator Edward Kennedy of Massachusetts to regain the Democratic presidential nomination, could not resist blaming this continuing hospital cost escalation on members of Congress who had not supported his hospital cost cap legislation. Those representatives in turn blamed hospitals for not honoring their commitments. As we shall see, the kind of inflation the hospitals were now experiencing resulted primarily from factors in the economy that were largely beyond the control of any voluntary or mandatory program.

The following graph indicates that the rate of increase in total hospital expenses from 1966, the first year of Medicare, through 1980 was well beyond the level that could have been anticipated when Congress passed P.L. 89–97 in 1965. Although Social Security Administration actuaries had reluctantly estimated that during the initial phases of the program hospital unit costs and aged utilization would increase more rapidly than in the past,[15] they had not anticipated that total hospital expenses would grow at a compound annual rate greater

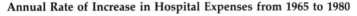

Annual Rate of Increase in Hospital Expenses from 1965 to 1980

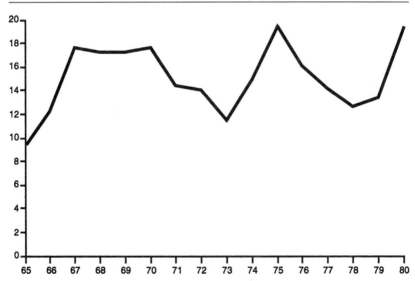

Source: American Hospital Association, *AHA Hospital Statistics*, 1991–92 and 1972 editions, for nonfederal short-term general hospitals.

than 15 percent over the program's first 15 years, with hospital expenses increasing from $9.1 billion in 1965 to $79 billion in 1980. Only in the third year of the Economic Stablization Program's controls, 1973, did the rate of increase in hospital expenses even remotely approach the pre-Medicare rates, and that was followed in 1975, the first-full year of decontrol, by an increase of 19.3 percent, a level that had not been reached since the years immediately after World War II.

As was cited earlier, Feldstein has persuasively argued that the underlying type of inflation in the hospital industry has been of the demand-pull variety caused by increasing demand stemming from a growing number of persons having low-dollar health insurance coverage. Medicare, by increasing insurance coverage for aged persons who were already heavy users of hospital services, even more significantly increased the demand for these services than the gradual expansion of coverage that had evolved through the sale of private health insurance. Hence, during the initial years of the program, hospital inflation resulted from a big spurt in demand-pull factors as increased health insurance coverage reduced the aged consumer's out-of-pocket cost for hospital services.

However, the 1975 and 1980 experiences contrast starkly with 1969 when 65.6 percent of the total increase in total hospital expense stemmed from increases in the quantity of inputs used to produce hospital services [McMahon and Drake 1978]. That pattern of cost increases resulting primarily from increased inputs is consistent with demand-pull inflation and the producer changing the nature of the product to meet the increased demand for services. The primary cause of hospital expense increases in 1975 and 1980 was, on the other hand, higher prices that hospitals had to pay for inputs and not larger quantities of inputs—73.3 and 78.8 percent of the hospital expense increases in 1975 and 1980, respectively, resulted from increases in factor prices [McMahon and Drake 1978 and Goldfarb et al 1982]. The cost-push increase in 1975 reflected postponed wage and supplier price increases from the 990 days of ESP that came due, and the 1980 cost-push increases were a consequence of the extremely high level of inflation in the general economy at that time, e.g., the Consumer Price Index rose 13.5 percent in 1980, and interest rates rose to 20 percent levels.

Although the peak increases of more than 19 percent in 1975 and 1980 were notable, the more serious problem was that the equilibrium rate of hospital expense growth had risen some 4 percentage points from about 10 percent in the pre-Medicare period to about 14 percent under Medicare. A 40 percent increase in the equilibrium rate of growth was the result of the expanded demand for hospital services by Medicare beneficiaries and possibly the reduced efficiency incentives inherent in the cost-recovery method of purchasing these services. In addition, the higher equilibrium rate of hospital expenditure growth also translated into the growth of total personal health expenditures to double-digit rates of increase, from an 8 percent rate of growth prior to Medicare to more than 12 percent in the 1970s.

The change in hospital utilization by the aged after the implementation was in large part responsible for the Medicare cost overruns. The rate of admission of those 65 and over had been expected to increase initially, and it did increase by 6.6 percent between 1965 and 1967. It simply continued to rise—45.9 percent between 1967 and 1980, or at an annual rate of slightly more than 2 percent. By 1980 the hospital was increasingly becoming a geriatric health care institution. When Medicare began in 1966, persons 65 and over had constituted slightly less than 10 percent of the U.S. population, about 20 percent of the admissions to short-term non-federal general hospitals, and about one-third of the total inpatient days. In 1980, the aged had grown to more than 11 percent of the population and represented 28 percent of hospital admissions and more than 41 percent of the total inpatient days.

The growth in the concentration of aged persons in the inpatient care market reflected higher inpatient utilization rates for the aged. Their inpatient admission rate rose 56 percent from 264 per 1,000 aged persons in 1965 to 411 in 1980. Inpatient utilization for the younger population virtually remained constant within a range of 125 per 1,000, the rate in 1965, and 130 when it peaked in 1980. The only documented inpatient utilization growth that occurred in short-term general hospitals after the implementation of the Medicare program was among aged persons, but it is possible that the disabled hospital rate also increased after 1973.

The effect of rising numbers of aged inpatients on the financing of acute inpatient care was twofold. First, the rate of increase in charges to the Medicare program was even higher than the rate of increase in hospital unit costs. From 1967 to 1980 the cost per hospital admission increased 3.9 times or at a rate of nearly 11 percent per year while annual admissions by aged persons nearly doubled from 5.337 in 1967 to 10.517 million in 1980. In cost accounting parlance, the volume variance, which reflected rising demand for hospital services among the aged population, was overwhelming the price variance, despite the magnitude of price increase. The overall result was a huge increase in Medicare expenditures, rising 7.8 times from $4.7 billion in 1967 to $36.8 billion in 1980 or nearly a 17 percent annual rate of increase [Gibson et al 1983].

Second, the federal government continued to change the accounting rules in its favor to pay a smaller portion of hospital costs per patient day. Therefore, as the number of Medicare days increased, the amount of the Medicare revenue shortfall increased. With fewer remaining private health insurance patients being hospitalized, the problem of cost shifting to a smaller patient base was becoming more acute for commercial insurance carriers and even some Blue Cross plans. Paradoxically, the smaller growth in the number of under 65 inpatients was producing higher (more than proportional) rates of increase in the prices hospitals had to charge private insurance patients in order to break even. Hospital charge structures lost any semblance of a relationship to the cost of providing services.

Neither the public nor the private sector could any longer afford to sustain the rapid rate of growth in hospital expenditures. At a minimum, fundamental changes in the method of paying for hospital services would be needed. The elimination of cost-recovery reimbursement would at least strengthen the hospital manager's incentives for cost containment. However, the more significant source of inflationary pressure, the proliferation of low-dollar hospital insurance, could not be changed so easily.

THE RISE OF THE PHYSICIAN ENTREPRENEUR

Government's efforts to restrain health care cost increases were not the only fundamental change in the health care market. In the mid to late 1970s the hospital-physician's 50 year-old noncompete alliance began to shatter under pressures from the excess resource capacities created by the Medicare-Medicaid programs and supplemented through the federal manpower grant programs. The scientific medicine complex had become so large that competition between its various components arose for the operating revenues necessary for their sustenance. Physicans started to unbundle services that had once been in the exclusive domain of the hospital. For the first time in this century, physicians formed specialized outpatient facilities to provide competing services, and hospitals began to lose health care market share. Surgicenters for ambulatory surgical services were the first type of physician-owned facilities that directly competed with hospitals. The first surgicenter was established in 1972 in Phoenix directly across the street from the flagship hospital of the Good Samaritan Health Care System. Developments in anesthesiology made it possible to perform a growning number of surgical procedures without general anesthesia. For these procedures it was no longer necessary to admit the patient to a hospital bed and require, at least, an overnight stay. The surgery could be performed in a single day without a costly hospital admission.

Renal Dialysis Centers—the New Prototype

However, both private health insurance carriers and the Medicare-Medicaid programs were reluctant, as collaborators in the old hospital-physician alliance, to cover services provided in these freestanding medical facilities. Surgery was not the first major service to move out of the hospital because patients were unwilling to pay for these procedures, even to gain its greater convenience. That honor fell to the new benefit that had been enacted as part of the 1972 Social Security Admendments—kidney dialysis for persons with end-stage renal disease. Three sites were available for dialysis depending on the patient's condition: in ascending order of cost, the patient's home, a freestanding ambulatory care facility, or the hospital's outpatient facility. Home dialysis is the least costly, but because of the initial startup costs for equipment, supplies, and training, the savings were not realized until the second year of treatment. For less severely ill patients, it may also be of higher quality and convenience. Obviously, the cost advantage of the home site will increase as treatment duration is extended [Delano et al 1981].

Dialysis service also was the first Medicare benefit to be paid for on a fixed national rate. During the '70s freestanding dialysis centers were paid $138 per treatment, and hospitals were offered the same rate but were permitted to charge up to 80 percent of their cost, which resulted in an average rate of $159 per dialysis treatment [Iglehart 1982]. There is evidence that hospital programs treated more severely ill patients [Plough et al 1984] to justify the higher rate. The maintenance of fixed rates for more than 10 years at the lower $138 price was sufficient to attract sizeable capital investment for more than 400 independent for-profit treatment centers by 1980. At that time, 600 hospitals were providing dialysis treatment facilities. The largest single provider was National Medical Care, which by 1980 had 60 facilities and had grown "from a $30 million-a-year enterprise in 1973 to a $245.5 million enterprise in 1980" [Iglehart 1982]. Although hospitals still treated more patients than the for-profit facilities in 1980, the independent centers and for-profit suppliers of continuous ambulatory peritoneal dialysis programs captured well over 70 percent of the dialysis market by the end of the 1980s.

A new prototype organization, which raised its capital as the investor-owned hospital systems had done, for entrepreneurial physicians had been created out of the entitlement for end-stage renal disease patients. It would soon be replicated for other formerly exclusive hospital services. Competition in the hospital industry was no longer just among hospitals. In the 1970s that competition increasingly came from physician entrepreneurs and hospital suppliers.

The success of ambulatory dialysis treatment guaranteed that other diagnostic and therapeutic services would be tested by other specialists wanting to become physician entrepreneurs. Changes in medical technology and knowledge, which had contributed so much to the initial growth of the hospital as the community's center for the practice of scientific medicine, now permitted some physician specialists to practice outside the hospital with manageable amounts of capital investment. The nephrologists were excellent market innovators in an expanding market in which their competition with hospitals benefited society by constraining unit treatment costs without doing serious economic injury to hospitals. Hospitals later gained revenues from other technology changes that permitted the successful transplantation of kidneys to provide more nearly complete cures for patients afflicted with renal failure instead of only the renal maintenance that dialysis provided.

The federal government's entitlement for end-stage renal disease proved to be much larger than estimated in 1972. The original estimates were that 10,000 first-year beneficiaries would increase to 90,000 by 1995 and then level off. That number was exceeded in the '80s, and recently it was estimated that the number of beneficiaries may

reach 300,000 by the end of the 20th century. The increase in beneficiaries stemmed largely from making dialysis available to older Americans than originally treated [Iglehart 1993 and Levinsky 1993].

Unraveling of the Hospital-Physician Alliance

Most of the growth in ambulatory care facilities outside the hospital
occurred during the 1980s. However, the seeds were sown in the
mid to late 1970s with small independent physician entrepreneurs
establishing diagnostic imaging, wellness/fitness, rehabilitation, urgent (primary), surgery, even birthing and other types of centers.
Perhaps the most visible centers in the early period were the urgent
care or emergicenters that were established in direct response to the
inconvenience and high unit cost of hospital emergency room services.
Hospitals had often complained about the financial responsibility of
operating 24-hour-a-day medical emergency services, which were often used for the treatment of minor ailments after physician office
hours. They found, however, that skimming off the less seriously ill
to the urgent care centers reduced the number of profitable patients
and increased the emergeny room's operating losses. Patients left the
emergency rooms for shorter waits and lower charges for care, even
with the addition of some allegedly unnecessary lab tests and x-rays
and occasional "true" emergencies that the centers were not equipped
to handle [Eisenberg 1980].

The increased supply of physicians accompanied by increased
specialization resulted in zero real growth in physicians' income during the 1970s and led to increased competiton among physicians for
patients and with hospitals for patient revenues. In total the physician-
population ratio rose from one practicing physician per 830 persons
in 1963 to one physician per 627 persons in 1980, or nearly a one-third
decrease in the number of potential patients per practicing doctor.
However, the growth in the number of primary care physicians (18.5
percent) over this 17-year period did not even keep pace with the 20.6
percent growth in the resident population. It was the 94.3 percent
growth in the number of surgical and other nonprimary care specialists
that created the greatest increase in competitive pressures among
physicians and between hospitals and doctors throughout the entire
country as the specialists came to practice increasingly outside metropolitan areas [McConnel and Tobias 1986].

As a consequence, physicians more frequently joined group practices with corporate legal organization, rather than partnerships. Freshnock and Jensen [1981] reported nearly a 70 percent increase in the number of medical group practices, a 220 percent growth in the number of physicians practicing in groups, and a shift in the percentage of groups organized as professional corporations from 15.6 percent in 1969 to 70.6 percent in 1980. Not only were there rising economic pressures for physicians to compete with hospitals for patient revenues, but the physician was increasing efforts to raise capital and, where possible, offer competing services.

The greatest potential economic threat for the hospital was ambulatory surgery because inpatient surgery produced nearly 50 percent of all hospital inpatient admissions. Even if hospitals were to counter the freestanding ambulatory surgery centers with their own outpatient surgery facilities, as they did, the loss of total hospital patient revenues was likely to be significant. However, just as with the dialysis centers, society would benefit from lower total health care costs because of the lower unit cost of outpatient surgical procedures.

The accommodation between hospitals and their medical staffs that had been made more than 60 years earlier was under great stress as more medical staff members had conflicts of interest with other staff members and with the hospital itself. When the Health Care Financing Administration and private health insurance companies granted coverage for services both in or out of the hospital, the old accommodation was no longer suitable to the 1980s. Some hospitals countered competition from members of their medical staffs by closing staff membership and employing economic as well as medical criteria for granting membership, called "economic credentialing" and subject to vigorous opposition by the AMA.

AN INDUSTRY UNDER SIEGE

Although health care providers had beaten off President Carter's simplistic effort to legislatively mandate an end to hospital cost increases, their prospects going into 1980 were not good. The industry's old anticompetitive alliances were beginning to break under the strain of too many hospital beds and too many physician specialists. A competitive virus was beginning to infect the industry. How this variety of competition would affect the battle over health care costs is the subject of the next chapter.

5

Provider Competition in an Era of Continuing Growth, 1980 to the Present

The second stage of the explosive growth phase in the health care industry began in the mid to late 1970s when the hospital-physician's 50-year-old noncompete alliance began to shatter under pressures from the excess resource capacities created by the Medicare-Medicaid programs and supplemented through the federal manpower grant programs. The scientific medicine complex had become so large that competition between its various components arose for the operating revenues necessary for their sustenance.

In addition to the rising number of physician specialists competing in the marketplace, two other changes had occurred. First, health insurance benefits were gradually extended to nonhospital-related ambulatory care. Second, technological changes, primarily in surgery, permitted many health care services to be provided outside the inpatient hospital for the first time since the scientific medicine revolution.

Although unit-price competition between the hospital and physician entrepreneurs was introduced to the health care industry, most consumers remained insensitive to price differences and made choices mainly on the basis of convenience and perceptions about the quality of the care. Therefore, the relative rate of health care inflation was virtually unaffected by these changes, but the growth of different sectors within the health care industry was modified. The hospital sector, because inpatient care was no longer as essential for the practice of scientific medicine as it had been, entered the mature phase of its development and lost market share to the physician sector and to comprehensive health care delivery organizations.

In the 1980s price competition had finally come to the health care market. The breakdown of the anticompetitive agreements that had dominated the market for so long occurred in the customary manner: it was no longer in the best economic interest of all parties to abide by the agreement. In this case, the physician specialists could no longer afford to restrict their practice of scientific medicine to the hospital. In order to increase their net return per patient contact in the increasingly crowded specialist market, specialists began to build their own diagnostic and therapeutic facilities outside the hospital to capture a larger share of the patient revenues.

This movement of patient services out of the hospital in turn created excess capacity in hospital facilities. With excess capacity in both the specialist physician and hospital markets, the private health insurers, who had been passive price-takers in the health care market-place for so long, could now more actively bargain on prices with providers. However, the initial bargaining was generally limited to unit prices, often in terms of discount from the list price of services. Never has so much been "saved" by so much spending! Unit-price competition not only developed naturally because of excess numbers of hospitals and doctors, but was also encouraged by a new type of broker or agent for employer-sponsors of health insurance plans that competed for "savings" with the more traditional health insurance companies.

Competition was limited to unit prices rather than the minimization of total health care costs because of the consumer's limited economic stake in the outcome. "Free" first-dollar health insurance coverage had grown to such an extent that the consumer was now making purchasing decisions without regard to the total cost of services. Purchasing agents were, consequently, limiting their role to minimizing unit costs. Just as there is good and bad cholesterol, there is good and bad competition. Unfortunately, unit-price competition was the bad kind of competition in that it really did not come to grips with the full measure of health care inflation.

With this overview of recent changes in the health care market, the chapter is organized to describe, in turn, their effects on the balance among health care providers, a revitalization of health insurers, and the continued passiveness of health care consumers.

SHIFTING BALANCE OF HEALTH CARE PROVIDERS

Cutting Hospitals with the Surgeons' Scalpels

The hospital's decline began in 1977 when short-term general hospitals started losing inpatient admissions in the under 65 age group. Total admissions and patient days for this age group continued, by and large, to grow slowly until 1981, when the admission and patient day rate per unit of population fell off even more rapidly at rates (2.9 and 4 percent respectively) exceeding the rate of growth in the number of persons 65 and over. By 1992 total inpatient admissions of those under 65 were only 81.4 percent, and nonaged patient days were about 70 percent of the 1981 totals.

Hospitals had previously experienced rapid rates of change in utilization, but until now the rates of change had always been positive—this was the first reduction in the demand for inpatient services that was not directly offset by increases from other groups of patients. For example, prior to the age of antibiotics in the 1930s, children were the second highest utilizers of inpatient services next to the aged. The growth in demand for hospital births allowed adult women to replace children whose reduced infection rates permanently reduced the demand for inpatient hospitalization among this age group.

Just as with children earlier, the reduction in the demand for inpatient care by nonaged adults reflected two changes in care technology. Although these changes were less significant than the discovery of antibiotics for reducing morbidity and mortality, the developments in surgery had the potential to be cost saving and to contribute to improvements in the quality of life. The first change related to the general development of localized anesthesia permitted surgery without the increased risks of debilitating and untoward effects of general anesthesia. Pragmatic surgeons rapidly adapted their techniques to a broad range of ambulatory procedures whenever localized anesthesia could be used. Same-day or short-stay surgery became the fastest-growing product line in health care, and surgery was no longer confined to inpatient hospitals.

Initially the under 65 age patients were the chief beneficiaries in terms of reduced surgical cost, loss of down time, and risk of injury or even death. The first outpatient surgeries were less invasive operations on the ear, eye, nose, mouth, pharynx, and female genital organs. However, the second change involved the development of the endoscope for examining internal organs through tiny incisions in the body. This led in mid-1988 to a whole new field of laparoscopic surgery that permitted surgeons to remove gallbladders, perform hysterectomies and tubal ligations, make hernia repairs, and even do appendectomies. Some have argued that laparoscopic surgery is not cost effective for the latter two procedures because of uncertainty about the enduring success of the hernia repairs and the relatively fast recovery time for the traditional appendectomy [Rosenthal, 1993 and Soper et al 1994]. By eliminating the usual wound required for abdominal surgery, laparoscopy has dramatically shortened the patient's recovery time and diminished postoperative discomfort.

Cataract surgery benefitted from the first change with localized anesthesia making it an ambulatory procedure. Because more older persons have cataracts, this procedure became the most frequent ambulatory surgery purchased by the Medicare program. However, many other outpatient procedures became available to the aged during the '80s. In 1983 the Health Care Financing Administration had approved some 450 procedures for payment in freestanding (physically separate from the hospital) ambulatory surgery centers (FASCs), and the number of approved procedures was 2,400 in 1992. As a consequence, the number of FASCs grew from 239 in 1983 to 1,556 in 1991 with only 7 percent being owned and operated by hospitals. The vast majority, 78 percent, were owned independently by physicians, physician groups, and other investors; and 15 percent were owned by corporate chains. The number of ambulatory surgery procedures purchased by the Medicare program rose from 377,000 in 1983 to 2.5 million in 1991 [PROPAC, June, 1993].

The effect on hospital utilization was dramatic, as Table 5.1 demonstrates. The number of surgical procedures performed (column 1) in hospitals continued to grow during this period. The rate of hospital surgery per the population (column 2) also continued to grow after falling off slightly in the early 1980s. However, by 1990 less than half of the hospital surgeries were done on an inpatient basis (column 3). Nevertheless, hospitals were able to attract half of their patient load for surgery (column 4), as measured by adjusted admissions, while surgery as a source of inpatients was plunging to less than one-third of its admissions.

Once the inpatient hospital was no longer the sole site of surgery, the genie was out of bottle and hospitals faced competition from physician entrepreneurs who organized surgicenters and other ambulatory care centers (including physician offices) in which surgery could

TABLE 5.1   The Number and Location of Hospital Surgical Procedures for 1980–1992

Year*	Millions of Procedures	Surgeries per 1,000	% Performed as Inpatient	Tot Sur/ Adj Adm*
1980	18.768	85.3	83.7%	45.3%
1981	19.237	85.9	81.5	46.1
1982	19.594	84.9	79.3	46.7
1983	19.845	84.5	76.2	47.6
1984	19.909	84.5	72.2	48.4
1985	20.113	84.1	65.4	50.2
1986	20.469	85.1	59.7	51.6
1987	20.817	86.8	56.2	52.8
1988	21.402	86.9	53.2	53.6
1989	21.340	86.6	51.5	53.2
1990	21.915	87.8	49.5	53.5
1991	22.405	88.8	47.7	53.7
1992	22.860	89.8	46.1	53.8

Source: American Hospital Association [1992]; AHA, *Hospital Statistics*, 1993–94; and U.S. Department of Commerce [1992]. Total surgeries as a percentage of adjusted admissions, is simply inpatient admissions adjusted for outpatient activities. The total output of a hospital is summarized by weighting the outpatient activies in terms of the relative amount of revenue generated and adding in/outpatient activity together.

be performed. Henderson [1992] has estimated that from 1984 to 1992 hospitals lost nearly 12 percent of the total surgery market through new procedures and patients moving to doctors' offices and ambulatory centers operated independently of hospitals. That is, he estimated that hospitals had 84.7 percent of the surgery market in 1984, but only 72.9 percent in 1992 in contrast to the American Hospital Association's estimates of nearly 91 percent in 1985 and 82.7 percent in 1990. Regardless of the magnitude, it is clear that surgery was a sizeable and growing activity outside of the hospital. At the same time the total number of hospital surgical procedures continued to increase, albeit with less inpatient activity.

Even though the inpatient hospital business was maturing, other sectors of the health care industry were still in the growth phase.

Both Henderson's and AHA's estimates of the hospital's penetration of the surgical market imply that the total number of surgical procedures in the United States in the last half of the 1980s and early 1990s increased about 20 percent every five years and that the rate of surgery per capita increased at more than 2 percent annually.

Certainly the technological advances in surgery, in terms of improved medical efficacy, lower unit costs, and increased patient convenience, overcame many of the impediments to having surgery. The unit cost per surgical procedure has dropped significantly through the reduction in inpatient stays, but that loss in revenues was being replaced by the increase in ambulatory surgical volume in which surgeons captured a larger percentage of the total revenue.

Maturity of the Inpatient Business

The engine, general acute inpatient care, that had driven the economic growth of the health care industry since the 1920s quit growing in 1981 when inpatient hospital capacity finally exceeded one million beds, admissions and patient days peaked at 36.5 million admissions and 277.4 million patient days, and hospital employment surpassed 4 million employees. Although the number of short-term general beds continued to grow slightly to 1,021,000 beds in 1983, this growth in inpatient capacity only contributed to falling hospital occupancy. Over these 53 years, the number of inpatient beds had almost exactly tripled from the 336,000 that Rorem had inventoried in 1928.

For the first time since the Great Depression the number of hospital closures after 1975 exceeded the number of new hospitals. The number of short-term general hospitals in the United States fell from 5,979 in 1975 to only 5,321 in 1992. That decline in the number of hospitals did not fully describe the decline in inpatient hospital utilization because the occupancy rate for the surviving institutions fell from almost 79 percent in 1969 to less than 66 percent in 1992.[16] Although hospitals continued to employ more than half of all health care personnel, 50.6 percent in 1993, that was a far cry from the two-thirds of all health care workers that hospitals had employed in the mid-1950s.

Nevertheless, the improvements in the inpatient hospital during its phenomenal expansion in the 20th century were spectacular. The greatest change among hospitals of all sizes was the investment in equipment and other capital facilities per available bed. Average investment in assets per bed in 1928 was $5,400 versus almost $96,000 in 1981, or adjusting for price level changes, a real growth in investment per bed of 3.5 times the 1928 level. Hospitals in 1981 were equipped for many services that did not even exist in 1928. The vast majority (70 percent or more) of general hospitals had ambulatory surgery, blood banks, diagnostic radioisotope, ultrasound, and physical and respiratory therapy. Close to a majority (40 percent or more) had CT scanners, histopathology labs, an organized outpatient department, and therapeutic radioisotope services. Close to 20 percent of the hospitals had nurseries for premature babies, hemodialysis facilities, and facilities for radioactive implants.

In order to operate all of these services, hospitals had to employ not only larger numbers of employees, but a higher proportion of very skilled, professional workers. The number of full-time employees per adjusted patient day rose from 2.24 in 1965 to 3.47 in 1981. However, hospitals were losing relative share in the health care labor market to home health care organizations, clinics, and HMOs. Their market share of health care spending peaked in 1982, when it reached 47.3 percent of personal health expenditures, and by 1991 had fallen to 43.7 percent. Hospitals had ceased to be the fastest growing sector in the health care industry. The decline began in 1977 when short-term general hospitals started losing inpatient admissions in the under 65 age group. By 1981 inpatient hospital admissions and patient days would cease to grow faster than the population for the first time in the 20th century.

As Table 5.2 indicates the final blow to the inpatient hospital business was the decline in utilization by the aged, which began falling rapidly in the early 1980s, but at a declining rate of of decrease. The growth in hospital utilization that took place in the first 10 or 11 years of the Medicare program gave the hospital what may be its final expansion. And, as was noted in chapter 4, that growth was largely generated by poor aged whose admission rate increased more than 2.5 times faster than the nonpoor [Kovar 1977]. Inpatient hospital services had reached the mature stage of business development in the classic fashion with the introduction of a lower-cost substitute. Outpatient services were becoming technologically available to replace the increasingly expensive inpatient hospital stay. As a result, hospitals were left with excess bed capacity that would finally permit price

TABLE 5.2   Inpatient Hospital Utilization by the Elderly for the Selected
Years 1965, 1977, 1987, and 1992

Year	Admissions per 1,000	Percentage Change	Patient Days per 1,000	Percentage Change
1965	264		3,447	
1977	362	37.1%	3,876	12.4%
1982	409	13.0	4,138	6.8
1987	353	(13.7)	3,133	(24.3)
1992	359	1.7	2,994	(4.4)

Source: The 1965 data are from DHEW [1977, 14 and the 1977, 1982, and 1987 are from
the AHA's National Hospital Panel Survey and U.S. Department of Commerce [1992].

competition to operate more effectively in the hospital industry even
without changing consumer incentives. Nevertheless, hospital unit
costs and revenues continued to increase so that total inpatient revenues and expenses would continue to rise, but real growth in the
number of inpatients served per capita would diminish after 1980.

Although the number of patient days had risen from 900 patient
days per 1,000 population in 1940 to 1,211 per 1,000 in 1980, a remarkable 33 percent increase in per capita utilization, and total inpatient
revenues had expanded by a factor of 87 or more than a 10 percent
per annum nominal growth rate, there was little progress in making
the hospital an integrated organization for the delivery or financing
of comprehensive health care services. The number of hospitals, inpatient beds, pieces of expensive equipment, and highly skilled employees had continued to grow. As a consequence, there were vast improvements in the quality and sophistication of hospital services.
However, the role of the hospital within the health care industry,
despite the growth in the hospital organization's size through the
creation of multihospital systems,[17] remained the physicians' workshop that had emerged by the 1920s.

Changing patterns of health insurance coverage, providing
greater parity between inpatient and outpatient coverage, and technological advances in medical practice had combined to end the eight
decades of tremendous growth in inpatient hospital revenues. Hospitals, if they were to continue to grow, would have to look for other
services to provide. The promise of hospitals becoming the integrating
nucleus for the development of a comprehensive health care organization has endured, at least in some markets and in the minds of many

other hospital executives. However, if a Clinton-like managed competition reform proposal is approved, it is more likely that most hospitals will play a lesser market role by becoming either a cost center in or a vendor for such a comprehensive delivery organization.

Competition and Medical Practice

While hospitals were struggling in the more competitive environment, physicians were experiencing substantial business expansion in the 1980s. Until 1982 the rate of change in spending on physician services tracked very closely with the change in the supply of practicing physicians. However, in the 10 years "since 1982, growth in spending on physician services has jumped 119 percent after inflation to $165.5 billion, while the number of doctors has increased just 34 percent" [Tully 1992].

As remarkable as the growth in outpatient surgery had been, the number of laboratory tests and X-rays billed to patients were each more than twice as frequent as the number of surgical procedures. Although these diagnostic procedures are much less expensive than surgery, the ability of third-party purchasers to validate the medical necessity is questionable, while computerized technology was proliferating the availability of tests and X-rays in clinics and doctors' offices. Because of the more than 30 percent growth in the number of practicing physicians in the 1980s, which was almost twice the rate of population growth of 18.6 percent, there was a need for physicians to maximize the revenue per patient seen by increasing the number of lab tests and X-rays provided in their offices or by referral to imaging or other diagnostic centers in which the physician has an ownership position.

Indeed, studies conducted by Mitchell and Scott [1992] of Florida physicians' referral patterns for physical therapy, Swedlow et al. [1992] of California referral patterns in workers' compensation cases, and Mitchell and Sunshine [1992] of referral patterns to jointly owned radiation theraphy centers in Florida all found significantly higher patient referrals and treatment costs when there was joint ownership of the facilities by the referring physicians. The U.S. Congress was concerned about the problem and has enacted tougher penalties for the Medicare and Medicaid "antikickback" provisions that were part of the 1972 Social Security Amendments. State governments are enacting tough prohibitions on physician ownership of facilities to which physicians might make self-referrals of patients [Mangan, 1993]. The American Medical Association's Council on Ethical and Judicial Affairs, which first attempted to remedy the conflict of interest through a mild disclosure proposal for dealing with the referral practices to jointly owned facilities, has condemned the joint ownership practice. The ethical dilemma for practicing physicians was not limited to outside facilities. The potential conflict of interest extended to large multispecialty clinics that increasingly have the facilities within their professional corporation to make self-referrals. The conflict also can extend to smaller groups where the technology permits many laboratory, surgical, and imaging services to be available on the practice premises. Although the AMA found that the separate ownership of therapeutic and diagnostic centers extended only to about 10 percent of the medical profession, the broader potential conflict of interest is much more pervasive with more medical care being practiced outside the hospital and its peer review activities.

Pope and Schneider [1992] "estimate that 42 percent of the growth from 1982 to 1988 in real net income per office-based physician was due to a greater number of services provided per physician, and the remaining 58 percent resulted from higher unit-profit margins." However, because of the substantially larger supply of physicians, they conclude that growth in the volume of services "accounted for two-thirds of aggregate income growth, while increased unit-profit margins explain only one-third."

The ease with which physician specialists could increase their incomes not only aggravated short-term rates of health care inflation, but it was undoubtedly responsible for an even more serious longer term dislocation in the health care market—the number of physician graduates from medical school were overwhelmingly (85 percent in 1991 and '92) choosing nonprimary care specilties because the income differential between primary and specialty care physicians had continued to widen. Pope and Scheider [1992] reported that "surgeons and medical specialists' income grew rapidly from 1982 to 1989 (by 33 percent and 31 percent, respectively), while general practitioners' average income was flat (only a 5 percent gain)."

Schroeder and Sandy [1993] contrast the U.S. distribution of physicians with other developed countries, where 50 to 70 percent of the physicans are generalists providing primary care. They conclude that specialty care "with its lavish use of the latest diagnostic and therapeutic techniques" is "a major reason health care consumed 14 percent of the gross national product in 1992, when in other developed countries—which depend much less on specialist physicians and their accompanying forms of technology—costs hovered around 8 percent. Our approach consumes resources in the health care sector that could perhaps be devoted to jobs, education, and infrastructure; even if these dollars remained in health care, they could be more wisely devoted to primary care, preventive services, and coordinated care for patients with chronic illnesses—activities that engender both better health and better quality of life."

THE RESURGENCE OF HEALTH INSURERS

While scientific medicines' penchant for high-tech, specialized care was growing outside the hospital, health insurers were trying to stop the rising tide by adopting more aggressive tactics in their war against health care inflation. The federal government, whose budget was hemorrhaging from rising health care costs, made a number of major interventions in attempts to control the bleeding. Private insurers soon followed with their own tactics.

The Revolution in Medicare

The spurt of excessive inpatient hospital inflation of 19.3 percent in 1980 had been the final straw for both congressional and administration officials; Medicare expenditures had risen by more than 20 percent that year. Even though the rate of hospital expense increases subsided somewhat in 1981 and '82 to 14.9 and 15.8 percent,[18] the Congress and the new Reagan Administration were committed to bringing hospital costs for the aged under control, something President Carter had been unable to do. However, President Reagan was also committed to not using regulatory controls to reach this objective.

This time hospital representatives knew that voluntary cost containment programs would hold no influence at either end of Pennsylvania Avenue—real changes in Medicare reimbursement were going to be made and, for the federal government, relatively quickly. Reagan's first budget hearings in 1981 for fiscal year 1982 were preoccupied with the tax and spending issues of the Reagan Revolution.

However, in 1982 Congress legislated a Carter-like cap on Medicare spending for hospitals in the Tax Equity and Fiscal Responsiblity Act (TEFRA) through target rate limits on total inpatient operating costs for the three fiscal years of 1983–85. Congress had provided an escape hatch for hospitals to avoid these limits if they could reach agreement with the Department of Health and Human Sevices on a legislative proposal for a fixed-price prospective payment system that would replace the retrospective cost recovery basis of payment. With the TEFRA limits acting like a gun at their heads to come to the bargaining table and establishing boundaries for the prospective payment negotiations, hospitals quickly accepted a prospective payment system (PPS) based on establishing prices for 467 admission categories labeled diagnosis-related groups (DRGs).[19]

Congress approved the Social Security Amendments of 1983 in May to implement PPS on October 1, 1983, and establish a new entity, the Professional Review Organization (PRO), to replace the Professional Standards Review organization and to review the medical necessity of hospital admissions for payment. Although the incentives of PPS were to minimize costs and earn profits by providing care at less than the prospective rate, there was concern that hospitals would also be encouraged to admit patients not requiring care as a means of increasing revenues with little cost effort. It was this concern about unnecessary admissions that led HHS to advocate the PRO process.

The new payment program's effect on inpatient care of Medicare beneficiaries must have exceeded the greatest expectations of the payment design experts in HHS. The biggest surprise, of course, was the large reduction in the admission rate of the elderly when an increase had been expected. That had been the reason for strengthening the utilization review process with the new PROs. However, that proved to be unnecessary because of changes in the number and type of physicians and HCFA regulatory changes. Almost simultaneously with the introduction of the PPS change in reimbursement, HCFA revised its policy concerning the acceptability of outpatient surgery in freestanding ambulatory surgery centers.

Although inpatient revenue had been diminishing in relative importance to outpatient revenue since the implementation of Medicare, it had only fallen from 91.5 percent of total patient revenue in 1967 to 86.7 percent in 1981. Even with the additional growth of outpatient revenue during the '80s, the economic success of the hospital would still be critically dependent on inpatient activities. Hospital inpatient occupancy dropped from 73.4 percent in 1983 to 64.2 percent in 1986 before it started to increase slightly. Consequently, hospitals' operating profits would also have dropped precipitously if HCFA had not chosen the role of benevolent oligopsonist and established the initial PPS rates at a quite generous level.[20]

Nevertheless, payments to hospitals for inpatient services dropped from an average annual increases of 13.1 percent for 1981–84 to an average increase of 2.4 percent for 1985–88. Clearly the change in reimbursement policy was important to the federal government's ability to control the budget for the Medicare trust fund. However, the reduction in the number of elderly hospital admissions provided a major assist in protecting the solvency of the Part A Medicare trust fund. The rate of increase in total Medicare expenditures continued in double digits through 1988 because the reduction in admissions had simply been surgical patients who had been transferred to the hospital's outpatient department or to physician-controlled FASCs, both Part B benefits. The 2.1 million increase in ambulatory surgery for the aged between 1983 and 1991 more than accounted for the reduction in aged inpatient hospital admissions over this eight-year period. It also explains why the rate of increase in the growth of Medicare program expenditures did not fall anywhere near as rapidly as the reduction in the elderly's inpatient utilization. The rate of increase in Medicare program expenditures, however, dropped from an average of 17.9 percent per annum in the eight years before the advent of PPS to 9.4 percent in the eight years after PPS's implementation.

The Medicare program failed to realize the full saving in the reduction of the rate of increase in hospital costs because of the off-setting increase in physician billing for ambulatory surgery in FASCs. Although the technological advances in surgery could be expected to increase the demand for surgery—it was a better, less costly product to the patient with the shorter recuperation and safer, more predictible outcomes, the rates of increase in particular procedures was phenomenal. For example, the Prospective Payment Assessment Commission (ProPAC), which was established in the 1983 legislation of PPS to independently evaluate the new payment system, reported that all of the following surgical procedures more than doubled between 1988 and 1990: diagnostic colonscopy; colonscopy, lesion removal; secondary cataract laser surgery; upper GI endoscopy biopsy; colonscopy and biopsy; and, kidney stone fragmentation [ProPAC, June 1993]. The 15 most common procedures, totalling 2.3 million in 1990, had increased in frequency some 76 percent in just two years; 6 of those 15 procedures were solely for diagnostic purposes, and these procedures constituted 41.7 percent of the 1990 total.

More Aggressive Purchasing Practices

Although some of the gains in health care cost containment were lost through the increase in ambulatory surgery, HCFA had finally broken the double-digit rate of increase in hospital costs, and for six consecutive years from 1984 through 1989 hospital cost increases were in the 6 to 9 percent range. The rate of increase in personal health expenses also fell to rates of increase of 8 or 9 percent during this six year period. In one year, 1984, the 8.4 percent of increase in personal health expenses was actually lower than the 10.9 increase in the U.S. gross domestic product. The respite was short lived, however, and the rate of increase in most of the health care cost indicators were back to the double-digit level in the 1990s.

Nevertheless, both federal and private purchasers of health care had seen enough favorable results in the '80s to press on with more aggressive purchasing practices. HCFA became the beneficient oligopsonist in the inpatient hospital market by setting its prospective DRG rates with an eye toward the overall financial status of hospitals because "continued access to hospital care for Medicare beneficiaries, Medicaid recipients, and others depends on hospitals' overall financial strength" [ProPAC 1993, 61]. The DRG rates can serve as a major determinant of hospital profitability and affect the level of cost shifting to the private sector, which in 1991 had reached a markup on cost for the average private sector purchaser of 31 percent [ProPAC 1993, 72].

It is appropriate for the Prospective Payment Assessment Commission to assume one of the traditional regulator's responsibilities for ensuring that the consumer is not injuried by the lack of available, safe, regulated products. The inpatient hospital is increasingly becoming a geriatric facility with the elderly constituting 37.3 percent of the admissions and 48.0 percent of the inpatient days in short-term community general hospitals in 1993, according to the National Hospital Panel Survey. In addition, capital payments have finally been incorporated into the Medicare prospective payment system so that hospitals are dependent on that system for both capital and operating payments.

In 1992, after congressional authorization in 1989 and a temporary freeze on physician fees, HCFA even took on the difficult assignment of trying to modify the physician fee structure by employing a resource-based relative-value scale (RBRVS) to increase payments to primary care physicians and reduce specialists' payments as a means of redressing the imbalance between the two types of physicians. It is too early to evaluate the new payment schedule, but the developers of RBRVS believe that the initial fee schedule "produces unreasonably low levels of payment overall, which could dissuade those considering a career in medicine from entering the field" [Hsiao et al 1993]. Even the Physician Payment Review Commission, the analogous agency for doctors to the hospital's ProPAC, expressed concerns as average physician fees for Medicare dropped from 68 percent of private fees in 1989 to an expected 59 percent of private fees in 1994 [Pear, 1994b].

With the federal government focusing in on administrative pricing systems for health care that emphasize its oligopsonist role, it is not surprising that private purchasers of care, primarily employer groups directly or brokers serving as their agents, would also seek to minimize their share of total health care costs by negotiating the best deal possible with health care providers. An increasing number of employers realized that experience rating put them at risk for the health care costs of their employees. The majority of all employer groups, and as many as 85 percent of groups with more than 5,000 employees, are self-insuring and contracting with Blue Cross, other private health carriers, or various brokerage organizations as third-party administrators of their self-insured plans [Iglehart 1992]. In addition to administering the plans, these new brokers also claim to be able to form provider groups that would offer lower prices for health care services.

These negotiated arrangements with health care providers are being called "managed care," which can encompass multiple and alternative functions. Initially managed care focused on changing programs to regulated patient-provider conduct, such as pre-admission testing before hospital admission, second opinions before surgery became qualified for insurance coverage, and required certification of days of hospital stay. By second guessing doctors and putting constant pressure on their fees, these programs left providers in a sea of paper and created a serious enmity between practicing physicians and third party purchasers of care. Physicians no longer billed patients, but instead learned to play billing games with these third parties.

The second phase of this contest took on an organizational emphasis. A survery by the Health Insurance Association of America reported that 47 percent of all employees in 1991 were enrolled in a managed care organization. The simplest new entity is the preferred provider organization (PPO), an organization that administers the plan and selectively contracts with fee-for-service providers based on discounted prices. The HMOs are the most complex managed care organizations in that they underwrite the health insurance risk for the employer and persuade health care providers to accept various degrees of that risk. Various types of HMOs have been established; network or independent practice associations (IPAs) forms of HMOs are groups or associations of physicians and independent hospitals that have contracted to provide health care on a capitation or other fixed-sum basis. Network or IPA HMOs were organized to lower the costs of care with a minimum of permanent restructuring by changing the payment incentives to providers to discourage unnecessary services while giving consumers the widest possible choice of physicians, the closest HMO option to full freedom of physician choice.

Although these new arrangements have obtained some savings for particular employer groups, the fastest rising cost components of personal health expenditures during the late '80s and early '90s were expenditures for program administration and the net cost of insurance, which rose between 15.6 and 16.6 percent annually from 1989 to 1991. All health care providers also experienced substantial increases in administrative expenses and levels of frustration during this period as they had to defend both prices and the appropriateness of specific patient procedures. Woolhandler et al [1993] have found that administrative expenses in hospitals had reached 24.8 percent of total hospital expenses in 1990 and argue that managed care competition is in large part responsible for these extremely high administrative expenses.

The limitation of unit-price competition can be observed in several market indications. First, in a competitive market that is working effectively there is normally only a small variance between actual prices and the competitive or equilibrium price. However, in the health care market the price variance appears to be increasing as more purchasing groups try to achieve market advantages over other groups. The excess supply of providers, specialists and hospital facilities, are playing a game of fictitious unit prices rather than competing on the basis of the total price of health care services. The quantity of services being sold by these health care providers is increasing or the identification of the services being provided is being changed to lessen the effects of the discounted unit price schedule on provider revenues.

The second indication is the level of provider income. During the 1970s when physician supply vis-à-vis the population first started growing, doctors' real income remained constant or dropped slightly. However, during the 1980s and thus far in the 1990s physician incomes are rising in real terms, i.e., the rate of increase in nominal income is greater than the rate of inflation. Hospitals have also reported average profit margins of about 5 percent in the last five years without any indication of worsening financial conditions in a supposedly more competitive market. However, earlier in the '80s short-term general hospitals had experienced the highest rates of institutional failure since the 1930s. Normally, economists would predict that physicians in excess supply would be unable to maintain real increases in net income and that hospitals with excess capacity should experience falling profit margins and continued closures.

The third indication is that the rate of increase in total health care costs continues its steady climb. After falling to single digit rates of increase from 1984 to 1989, personal health expenditures grew at rates of 10.5, 12.8, and 12.9 percent from 1990 to 1992, and total national health expenditures continued to grow faster than the U.S. gross domestic product by reaching 14 percent in 1992. Even with the six years of single digit health care inflation in the '80s for the first time since 1965, over the decade of the 1980s, "whether in absolute dollar terms or relative to its GDP, U.S. health expenditures have increased faster than spending in other [developed] countries, and the gap between the United States and other major industralized countries have increased" [Schieber et al 1992].

In light of the continuing escalation of U.S. health care costs, it may well be that the effects of many of these managed care organizations are only cosmetic. The only exceptions may be the staff model HMOs (in which physicians are employed) and the closed panel group practice HMOs. In these two types of HMOs the care payment incentives to providers are reversed from providing more to doing less, and these organization have many more primary care physicians than specialists compared to the general marketplace and fewer inpatient beds by far than the ratio of beds to the general population. These two kinds of HMOs reflect the payment incentive to substitute primary and ambulatory care for the specialist, high technology care being provided in the rest of U.S. health care market. These organizations compete on the basis of total health care price, not on fictitious unit prices. Rice, Brown, and Wyn [1993] have concluded that much of the HMO growth (about 60 percent) has been in networks or IPAs that have produced little evidence of cost savings over the conventional fee-for-service health care delivery system.

PASSIVE HEALTH CARE CONSUMERS

Without the active support of health care consumers, the best efforts of health insurers or, for that matter, health care regulators to control costs is doomed to failure in a free market economy. Recent consumer responses to changes in relative prices of health care services demonstrate that price changes will affect consumer behavior, even when the prices to the consumers are totally unrelated to the cost of providing those services.

Consumers Respond to Artificial Prices

At the same time physicians were seeking to provide more outpatient services, the consumer received substantial price reductions through the extension of health insurance coverage to outpatient care. Table 5.3 presents a summary of the sources of financing personal health services for the 26 years between 1965 and 1991, in five-year increments from 1965 to 1980 and then yearly. The first increases in the share of personal health expenditures financed through private health insurance took place during this period. Because Medicare took over responsibility as primary carrier for those 65 and over, the insurance carriers' share dropped in the first five years and then increased in the 1970–75 period, probably as a result of Medigap policies that were sold to the aged.

Medicare was the first health insurance program to reduce consumer out-of-pocket expenditures for both hospital and physician services.[21] Part B of Medicare, the voluntary medical coverage, substantially reduced the average percentage of consumer out-of-pocket expense to the total medical bill by some 15 percentage points in the interval between 1965 and 1970, while private insurance picked up an additional 2.8 percentage points, largely through Medigap coverage for the elderly. The additional portion of the physician bill that was paid by Medicare probably resulted from the addition of the disabled as Medicare beneficiaries in 1973 and an increase in the number of

TABLE 5.3 Personal Health Expenditures by Source of Funding for Selected Years between 1965–1991

Year	Personal Health Expenditures		Consumer out-of-pocket			Private Health Insurance			Government		
	$ Spt*	% Chg**	$ Spt*	% Chg**	% Tot***	$ Spt*	% Chg**	% Tot***	$ Spt*	% Chg**	% Tot***
1965	$ 35.6		$ 19.0		53.4%	$ 8.7		24.4%	$ 7.3		20.5%
1970	64.9	14.4%	25.6	2.9%	39.4	15.2	11.7%	23.4	22.4	25.2%	34.5
1975	116.6	12.6	38.5	8.5	33.0	29.9	14.5	25.6	45.3	15.2	38.9
1980	219.4	13.4	59.5	9.1	27.1	65.3	16.9	29.8	87.1	13.7	39.7
1981	254.8	16.1	67.2	12.9	26.7	77.1	18.1	30.3	101.6	16.6	39.9
1982	286.4	12.4	74.2	10.4	25.9	88.5	14.7	30.9	113.5	11.7	39.6
1983	314.9	10.0	81.4	9.7	25.8	97.3	9.9	30.9	125.3	10.4	39.8
1984	341.2	8.4	87.7	7.7	25.7	106.3	9.2	31.2	135.7	8.3	39.8
1985	369.7	8.4	94.4	7.7	25.5	114.0	7.2	30.8	148.4	9.4	40.1
1986	400.8	8.4	100.9	6.9	25.2	123.8	8.6	30.9	162.1	9.2	40.4
1987	439.3	9.6	108.8	7.8	24.8	137.7	11.2	31.3	177.8	9.6	40.5
1988	482.8	9.9	119.3	9.7	24.7	154.1	11.9	31.9	192.6	8.3	39.9
1989	529.9	9.7	126.1	5.7	23.8	169.6	10.1	32.0	215.2	11.7	40.6
1990	585.3	10.5	136.1	7.9	23.3	186.1	9.7	31.8	241.8	12.4	41.3
1991	660.2	12.8	144.3	6.0	21.9	222.2	19.4	33.7	285.1	17.9	43.2

Source: Levit et al 1991 and the Office of National Cost Estimates 1990.

Personal Health Expenditures:
    * Dollars Spent (in Billions)
   ** (Annual) Percentage Change
Consumer Out-of-Pocket
  *** Percentage of Total (Personal Health Expenditures)
    Private Health Insurance (Expenditures)

physicians who accepted Medicare allowable charges as full payment for their services (technically called "accepting assignment") in the late 1980s and early '90s. In any event, Medicare ended up paying another 8.3 percentage points of the average physician's bill from 1970 to 1992.

Higher consumer out-of-pocket payments for physician services than for hospital services had been the pattern, in large part because of the insistence of the American Medical Association that medical coverage be limited to physician services that were hospital related, principally for surgical services. Once Medicare had changed this pattern, private health insurance followed and assumed a higher share of the nonaged consumer's share of the physician's bill, another 12.7 percentage points. These coverage changes were introduced with the expectation that nonhospital related physician benefits would reduce the consumer's incentive to seek inpatient care by substituting ambulatory services.

By 1990 private health insurance, which had been created in the 1930s to insure against the high cost of hospital care, was paying a greater percentage of the physician's bill, 45.2 percent, than any other payment source. Private health insurance only paid 36.5 percent of the hospital bill, but because hospital expenses were nearly $100 billion more than expenses for physician services, the insurers made $23.1 billion more in hospital payments than in payments to physicians. Government programs were picking up the majority, 54.1 percent, of the nation's hospital expenses. Government became the principal purchaser of hospital services because its beneficiaries—the poor, the aged, the disabled, veterans, and other wards of the state—were the heaviest utilizers of hospital services even though they did not represent a numerical majority of Americans.

Table 5.4 provides the same source of funding information for physician services that table 5.3 provides for spending on all health care services. It shows that the net effect of new health insurance programs and benefits was to reduce the consumer's share of the bill for physician services by about two-thirds in the 25 years from 1965 to 1990, from 62.6 percent to 20.7 percent of the total. Despite a tenfold increase in expenditures for physican services in this quarter of a century, the consumer's out-of-pocket expenditures did not even double, going from $3.3 billion in 1965 to $5.7 billion in 1990. In contrast, consumer out-of-pocket expenditures for hospital care, in spite of a much lower cost sharing ratio (4 percent versus 20 percent

TABLE 5.4   Source of Financing Physician Services* for Selected Years between 1965–1990

Year	Consumer	Private Insurance	Government	Total Expenditures	Annual % Chg.
1965	62.6%	29.7%	7.7%	$ 9.1	9.1%
1970	44.4	32.5	22.5	15.1	10.5
1975	34.7	36.2	27.6	26.8	12.2
1980	29.8	39.9	28.3	50.6	13.1
1985	24.5	42.9	30.2	90.6	12.3
1990	20.7	45.2	31.8	159.6	12.1

Source: Suzanne W. Letsch et al [1992] and the Office of National Cost Estimates [1990]. *Physician services are defined as the categories of direct expenses of physicians and of other professional services because the latter services include outpatient clinics and freestanding dialysis centers; see the latter referenced source for a complete definition.

for physician services), almost quadrupled from $2.8 billion in 1965 to $10.3 billion in 1990.

The relative cost to the consumer of physician services fell in real terms, i.e., adjusted for inflation, and vis-à-vis competing hospital services. It is small wonder that the nation was able to absorb a doubling of the number of practicing physicians between 1965 and 1990 without reduced relative earnings by physicians. Based on the most rudimentary conformance with the law of supply and demand, consumers were willing to purchase many more physicians services with such a substantial "price" decrease, and physicians were able to maintain and even to increase their total income because private health insurance and the government paid much higher prices. Needless to say, the hospital's penetration in the health care market, as measured by percent of health care spending, fell from 47.3 percent in 1982, when it reached its zenith, to 43.6 in 1990. During this same 8-year period, physician services grew from 24.5 percent of personal health care services to 27 percent.

Consumer Apathy About "Real" Health Care Prices

Unfortunately, in the current health care marketplace even the staff or closed panel HMO will have a difficult job selling more efficient health care because the primary decision maker for health care purchasing does not care about price competition in the health care market. The consumer's decisions are not based on real prices because employer-provided health insurance benefits have negated the normal consumer decision-making process at point of service.

The average consumer has been much less concerned about the price of health care since the implementation of Medicare in 1966. As Table 5.5 shows, health care expenditures over this 35-year period have fallen rapidly as a percentage of personal health expenditures from 64.5 percent in 1965 to 38.4 percent in 1990, column 3. Out-of-pocket expenditures by consumers at the time personal health care services are obtained have fallen even more substantially from 53.1 percent in 1965 to 23.3 percent in 1990, column 4. Since 1965 the only consumer payments for health care that have increased as a percentage of personal health care expenditures are the Medicare Part B insurance premiums and the Medicare payroll tax, which has risen from a combined 5.1 percent in 1970 to 7.8 percent in 1990, columns 6 and 7. The only type of consumer payment that has been a relatively stable percentage of personal health expenditures is the 7.1 to 7.7 percent, column 5, spent by consumers on private health insurance premiums since 1970. That percentage dropped from 11.5 percent in 1965 because the aged substantially reduced their private premiums when Medicare coverage became available.

TABLE 5.5 Type of Consumer Expenditures on Health Care for Selected Years between 1965–1990

Year	Personal Health Exp*	Consumer Payments**	% Total	Out-of Pocket as % Tot	Insurance Premium as % Tot	Medicare Premium as % Tot	Medicare Tax as % Tot
1965	$ 35.8	$ 23.1	64.5%	53.1%	11.5%	—	—
1970	64.9	33.6	51.8	39.4	7.1	1.5	3.6%
1975	116.6	54.9	47.1	33.0	7.6	1.5	4.9
1980	219.4	90.3	41.2	27.1	7.4	1.2	5.5
1985	369.7	152.0	41.1	25.5	7.7	1.4	6.5
1990	585.3	224.7	38.4	23.3	7.3	1.7	6.1

Source: Iglehart [1992] from Health Care Financing Administration data. Because of rounding, not all total percentages add to 100 percent, and the figure for personal health expenditures in 1965 is slightly different from the number used elsewhere in the text.

*Personal Health Expenditures (in billions)
**(Total) Consumer Payments (in billions)

When consumer expenditures for health care over this period are compared to personal (before taxes) or disposable (after taxes) income, as they are in Table 5.6, it is clear that the level of consumer health care expenditures has nearly kept pace with increases in personal income, except for the increase in Medicare taxes. On an after-tax basis, the average consumer is spending slightly less, 4.8 percent in 1965 and only 4.7 percent in 1990. There has been no significant increase in health care costs as far as the average consumer's percent of income is concerned even though the nation as a whole is devoting more than twice as much of its gross domestic product for health care than it was in 1965, 5.9 percent versus 12.2 percent in 1990.

The consumer's insulation from the direct effect of health care costs cancels out most signals or incentives for changing health care consumption. Nevertheless, the decrease in the relative cost of ambulatory care vis-à-vis inpatient care as ambulatory insurance coverage expanded in the 1980s did encourage consumers to modify their behavior because their out-of-pocket cost for outpatient care was reduced both in absolute dollars of cash cost and relative to the cash cost of inpatient care. However, this change in the relative cost of unit prices actually worked against consumers joining HMOs because a previous advantage of HMOs over the traditional fee-for-service delivery system was that HMOs charged much lower fees at the time of service for their ambulatory services than the schedule of copayments for fee-for-service health insurance policies.

In addition, and perhaps more significant, the consumer has little incentive to compare the overall cost of care in the à la carte, fee-

TABLE 5.6   Consumer Health Care Spending as a Percentage of Income for Selected Years between 1965–1990

Year*	Consumer Health Expend (CHE)	Personal Income (PI)	CHE As % PI	CHE − Health Taxes	Disposable Personal Income (DPI)	CHE − Taxes As % DPI
1965	$ 23.1	$ 552.9	4.2%	$ 23.1	$ 491.0	4.8%
1970	33.6	831.0	4.0	31.2	722.0	4.7
1975	54.9	1,307.3	4.2	49.2	1,150.9	4.3
1980	90.3	2,264.4	4.0	78.3	1,952.9	4.0
1985	152.0	3,379.8	4.5	128.0	2,943.0	4.3
1990	224.7	4,664.2	4.8	189.0	4,042.9	4.7

Source: Iglehart [1992] and Council of Economic Advisers [1993].

for-service system with the premium cost of an HMO, or to compare premium differences between an IPA type HMO and a closed panel group HMO. Consequently, with the diminution in importance of comparative premium costs, the consumer's decision is likely to be based on the relative benefits, and a closed-panel HMO is at a disadvantage to fee-for-service health insurance and network or IPA HMOs because of the reduced choice of physicians in the closed panel model. Greater total cost savings are not part of the trade-offs that most consumers consider in choosing either their type of health insurance or HMO coverage.

With the reduced importance of total premium cost for consumers, it can be expected that different kinds of HMOs, even those that are organized for greater cost savings, will also tend to compete for subscribers on the basis of superior, more convenient health care services at lower out-of-pocket costs. The recent decision by Kaiser Permanente, the nation's largest and most successful closed panel group practice HMO, "of giving enrollees the option of receiving services from non-Kaiser physicians," the so-called point of service option, is evidence of how the consumer's out-of-pocket prices for services will be able to erode the producer incentive for lower total cost health care services [Kenkel 1993]. Unless there is consistency of objectives between the demand and supply sides of the health care market, there cannot be effective price competition.

The consumer's disregard of total cost is the deficiency of unit-price competition, which in the 1990s health care market enables health care providers and health insurers to avoid the full rigors of price competition in the health care industry. Only employers, who have been bearing nearly all the premium costs of health insurance or HMO capitation rates, have any incentive to control total health care costs for their employees as a means of controlling fringe benefit costs and the total wage bill. Their options are the elimination of employee coverage or reduced employee choice of health benefits at the risk of reduced worker productivity resulting from increased employee discontent and labor disputes.

STATE OF THE HEALTH CARE MARKETPLACE

As health care in the United States approaches its centennial in the marketplace, some vestiges of the past market successes of scientific medicine are disappearing. The extraordinary rate of health care cost increases in the Medicare era coupled with excess capacity for scientific medicine in the overspecialization of U.S. physicians and hospital facilities has finally created a crack in the anticompetitive alliances of doctors and hospitals. However, only the inpatient hospital has reached the mature stage of market development with its implication for reduced growth or, in some markets, even for decline. The rest of the industry, including the hospital's outpatient services, are continuing to grow at only slightly less spectacular rates because a flawed health insurance financing mechanism keeps the money flowing to health care providers whose only binding market constraint is consumer sensitivity to the unit prices charged through out-of-pocket costs or discounted unit prices contracted with the brokers of employer groups.

The integrated, comprehensive health care delivery and financing organization that economic development in other industries would have predicted has made some progress during the last quarter century, but it still competes at a disadvantage in the current marketplace, especially in terms of its potential for minimization of health care costs. The overarching conclusion is that market reform is vitally needed in the health care industry. Only a major restructuring, which must include the federal government's participation can overcome the health care market's failures. However, past government activities in this marketplace do not offer much hope that successful market reform is at hand.

6

The Retrospective on the Health Care Industry: What Went Wrong and Why

Agreeing that the health care market is broken and needs fixing is only a preliminary step in constructing a health care reform proposal for the United States. Now the more difficult assignment is to analyze the more than 90 years of U.S. health care market experience and to identify specifically what went wrong and why. Only then can the characteristics of an effective reform proposal be crafted. Two dimensions of the U.S. health care system are critical: its organization of health care resources and its composition as a marketplace.

Concerning the organization of health care resources, the study has found that the early advocates of scientific medicine have been too successful in competing with other segments of the medical profession in the design and operation of the delivery system. Initially the scientific school of medicine actively pursued a set of objectives for creating a health care delivery system that stressed a disciplined science and technology approach to care. By the 1930s that school became politically inactive and simply permitted the GPs' impulsive reactions and the popularity of their achievements to solidify their gains in the post-World War II development of the industry. Although the success of this school is not a flaw in the health care market but rather the result of a market flaw, it represents a major finding of the study that suggests that there has been an overinvestment in science and technology in the United States. The first part of this chapter will confirm this diagnosis by comparing the U.S. health care delivery system with the delivery systems in other developed nations.

The second part of the chapter will analyze the more technical market characteristics of the U.S. health care financing and delivery system. However, the international comparisons will prove useful in focusing on the specific time that the success of the scientific school of medicine finally overstepped the bounds of reasonableness and the health care market went out of balance. Knowing when the market failed provides vital clues to the key market relationships that need fixing and thus are important to the success of health care reform.

OVERINVESTMENT IN SCIENCE AND TECHNOLOGY

An Overview of Health Care Systems

The most convincing evidence that the health care industry in the United States has overinvested in scientific medicine can be seen by comparing the U.S. investment with that of other developed nations. Data for such comparisons have recently become available from the Organization for Economic Cooperation and Development (OECD), which has collected, as uniformly as possible, information on health expenditures, utilization and availability of health care resources, and health status indicators for 24 member nations. Seven of these 24 nations—Canada, France, Germany, Japan, Sweden, United Kingdom, and United States—have been compared to show that the United States has overinvested in science and technology. The results would not have been affected by the inclusion of any or all of the remaining 17 OECD member. These seven nations were chosen because they exemplify both high and low styles of resource utilization, have been the subjects of a substantial amount of health services research, and are all major trading competitors or cultural partners of the United States.

Even the most casual comparisons of national health care delivery and financing systems reveal great diversity in organizing and financing health care and substantial latitude in the consumption of health care resources. Consumption is best measured in terms of the amount of resources allocated to health care out of the total quantity of resources produced in the economy for domestic use, the country's gross domestic product (GDP). There is nothing wrong per se with a nation consuming more of particular goods and services than other nations as long as the increased consumption reflects the tastes and preferences of that nation. However, the increase in health care con-

TABLE 6.1   Seven Developed Nations' Allocation for Health Care for Selected Years between 1960–1990

Country	1960	1965	1970	1975	1980	1985	1990
Canada	5.5%	6.0%	7.1%	7.2%	7.4%	8.5%	9.3%
France	4.2%	5.2%	5.8%	7.0%	7.6%	8.5%	8.8%
Germany	4.8%	5.1%	5.9%	8.1%	8.4%	8.7%	8.1%
Japan	2.9%	4.3%	4.4%	5.5%	6.4%	6.5%	6.5%
Sweden	4.7%	5.6%	7.2%	7.9%	9.4%	8.8%	8.6%
U.K.	3.9%	4.1%	4.5%	5.4%	6.0%	6.0%	6.2%
U.S.	5.3%	5.9%	7.4%	8.3%	9.2%	10.2%	12.1%

Source: As defined by the percentage of gross domestic product consumed for total health expenditures according to Schieber et al [1992].

sumption in the United States does not necessarily support any increased preference for buying more health care services by Americans. Spending cannot be equated with demand for services in a failed market. Table 6.1 presents the percentage of resources allocated for health care services by the seven nations for five-year intervals from 1960 to 1990.

Although the United States did not begin the period as the most profligate health care spender, since the implementation of the Medicare and Medicaid programs, the U.S. has devoted more of its GDP to health care than any nation in the world except in 1980 when Sweden briefly held that title. Furthermore, since 1970, and especially in the 1980s, the percentage by which the United States has exceeded even the second highest spender has been rising. In 1990 with 12.1 percent of its GDP being devoted to health care, the United States allocated 30 percent more of its GDP to health care spending than the second highest nation, Canada. Over the entire 30-year period the United States increased its share of GDP for health expenditures more than any other country, and in the last decade of the 1980s that disparity grew at the most rapid rate. The problem of excess spending on health care in comparison to other developed nations is getting worse, not better.

The health spending experiences of other countries, however, offer some hope for being able to reverse the ever rising health care apportionment. Germany reduced its allocation from 8.8 percent in 1985 to 8.1 percent in 1990, and Sweden dropped from 9.4 percent in 1980 to 8.6 percent in 1990. These reductions demonstrate that a country can reduce its share of GDP devoted to health care expenditures and thus make available more resources for other, nonhealth goods and services.

Japan and the United Kingdom have maintained their allocations for health care at very low levels relative to the other developed nations. Japan has increased its health care allocation by more than 220 percent over the 30 years (almost as much as America's 224 percent), while only allocating 6.5 percent of its GDP to health in 1990. The United Kingdom increased its share by the smallest percent of the seven nations, 159 percent over the 30 years, and made the smallest allocation in 1990 of 6.2 percent of its GDP.

The data in Table 6.1 indicate that the United States spends more on health care by a substantial margin. However, the experience of Germany and Sweden suggests that this does not have to continue. Before exploring some of the possible approaches for the United States to reduce its health care costs, it is important to ascertain whether the United States obtains some benefits for its citizens by allocating 30 to 95 percent more of its GDP to health care than other developed nations.

Table 6.2 also used OECD data to compare the health status of citizens of these seven countries. The basic finding is that the United States has not achieved any major improvement in the health of Americans by allocating so much more of its resources to health care than other developed nations. In 1988 the United States ranked seventh of the seven nations in infant mortality, sixth in female life expectancy

TABLE 6.2   Seven Developed Nations' Health Outcome Indicators for 1988

Country	Infant Morality per 1,000	Female Life Expectancy (at birth)	Male Life Expectancy (at birth)	Female Life Expectancy (at age 80)	Male Life Expectancy (at age 80)
Canada	7.2	79.7	73.0	8.9	6.9
France	7.7	80.6	72.3	7.5	6.1
Germany	7.6	78.4	71.8	7.6	6.1
Japan	4.8	81.3	75.5	8.4	6.9
Sweden	5.8	80.0	74.2	8.1	6.3
U.K.	9.0	78.1	72.4	8.1	6.4
U.S.	10.0	78.3	71.5	8.7	6.9

Source: Schieber et al [1991].

at birth, fourth in male life expectancy at birth, second in female life expectancy at 80, and was in a three-way tie for first in male life expectancy at 80. This is certainly not an extraordinary record of accomplishment. Except for infant mortality and male life expectancy at birth, the United States has been able to exceed somewhat the health status indicators of the United Kingdom, but at almost twice the relative level of spending. On the other hand, Japan has better or equal health indicators than the United States in every category except female life expectancy at 80—and it only allocates 54 percent as much of the Japanese GDP for health care as the U.S., 6.5 percent for Japan versus 12.1 for the United States.

Even though the United States has not obtained good value for its very large allocation of resources for health care, some American health spending programs have contributed to better health for some Americans. As was noted in chapter 4, there was a substantial reduction in infant mortality and an increase in the life expectancy of aged Americans after the implementation of the Medicaid and Medicare programs in 1966, and the OECD data reflect a relative improvement in the U.S. standings through the end of the 1970s. No other remarkable findings were evident for the entire 30-year period that are not demonstrated in the 1988 comparisons in Table 6.2.

It is not surprising that the health status indicators do not reflect significant benefits because health status depends upon many factors other than health care [Belloc and Breslow 1972 and Breslow 1978]. For example, almost two-thirds of the U.S. reduction in age-adjusted mortality rates in the 1970s, and 98 percent of the mortality rate improvement in the 1980s, stemmed from a reduction in the death rate from major cardiovascular disease. Although the U.S. health care system made great technological progress in coronary care in this period, it is generally believed that changes in the life-styles of Americans—better nutrition, more exercise, and less smoking—were as, or perhaps even more, important to this improvement in our health.

Because health care is only one of the factors affecting health, we need to focus on the other reasons for the higher American health care costs. One reason often cited is that other developed countries have created national governmental financing systems that permit greater control of health care costs. It certainly is true that the United States pays a much lower percentage of its health care costs through public finances. In the seven-country comparison, governmental financing sources in the United States paid only 42 percent of the total health care bill in 1990. In the other six countries, government sources financed, on average, 78 percent of the total. Sweden was highest with 90 percent, and Japan was lowest with 72 percent public financing [Schieber et al 1992]. In one of the most thorough studies based on comparisons of national health care systems (in this case, Britain, France, Sweden, and the United States), Hollingsworth, Hage, and Hanneman [1990] concluded, "Historically, state funding leads to state involvement in many aspects of medical delivery systems and eventually to greater control over prices and personnel." In fact, Hollingsworth et al find few redeeming features in a nonpublic health care system except that these systems are "less rigid than state-managed systems, and they tend to provide a higher quality of care for upper-income groups."

Whether the historical relationship between greater public financing and better cost containment capabilities is applicable to the United States today may depend on the nature of the U.S. health care cost problem. If the problem is simply outrageously high fees, then greater government involvement could well be effective in reducing health care costs. If, however, the source of the U.S. health care system's inefficiencies is more complex, then greater bureaucratic control may be less effective. In any event, it will be useful to analyse the other differences between the U.S. health care system and the systems in these six developed nations.

Identifying the Cost Differences

The way different countries allocate their health care spending may prove illuminating. Table 6.3 has been prepared from OECD data that have been disaggregated by Dale A. Rublee and Markus Schneider [1991] to show how the seven nations' per capita health care spending was allocated. There may be some problems with the Rublee-Schneider disaggregation methodology (see Schieber-Poullier [1991]), but nothing that should diminish the data's usefulness in pointing out the nature of the U.S. cost problem. In calculating total per capita expenditures, Rublee and Schneider excluded the categories of research and development, construction, and administrative expenditures; i.e., they have used personal rather than total health expenditures.

TABLE 6.3   Seven Developed Nations' Allocation of Personal Health
Expenditures For 1988

Type*	Canada	France	Germany	Japan	Sweden	U.K.	U.S.
Hospital	48%	46%	34%	33%	47%	47%	43%
Physician**	11%	16%	16%	16%	10%	14%	21%
Drugs	12%	17%	17%	17%	7%	14%	8%
LT Care	12%	5%	8%	11%	16%	13%	10%
Dental	6%	7%	13%	6%	6%	4%	6%
Appliances	4%	4%	7%	5%	4%	2%	4%
Other	7%	5%	5%	13%	10%	6%	8%
Per Capita Expenditures	$1,495	$1,154	$1,200	$989	$1,389	$858	$2,006
% of U.S.	75%	58%	60%	49%	66%	43%	100%

Source: Rublee and Schneider [1991].
*Rublee and Schneider define the types of expenditure as follows: hospital expenditures
include acute, psychiatric, and long-term care and drugs provided in the hospital;
physician expenditures include ambulatory care of general practitioners in offices and
in outpatient departments of hospitals; drugs include both over-the-counter and prescription drugs that are provided outside of hospitals; long-term (LT) care includes
nursing home and home care expenditures; dental includes expenditures for therapeutic
and preventive care; appliances include glasses, hearing aids, medical equipment for
domestic use, and physiotherapy expenditures; and other expenditures include public
health, transportation, psychotherapy, and alternative medicine services.
**In the data on U.S. personal health care expenditures presented in the previous
chapters, the physican category of expenditures has also included "other professional"
expenditures to capture physician activities in clinics and other ambulatory care facilities.

Although the U.S. fared somewhat better in comparison to the
costs of the other six countries by the exclusion of administrative costs
for government and insurance programs, which are especially high
in the United States, U.S. costs per capita were still more than double
the Japanese and British rates and were one-third higher than the
next highest-cost nation, Canada. There were numerous reported
differences in the pattern of health care spending, such as the low
level of drug expenditures for the United States and Sweden (probably
due to the inclusion of hospital-administered drugs in the hospital
category). The substantial difference in the use of long-term care in
Sweden (16 percent of total expenditures) and in France (only 5 percent) was probably because 30 percent more of Sweden's population

was aged and it has a governmental system of nursing homes. The high level of dental expenditures in Germany reflects a higher fee schedule for dentists than physicians and the lack of a water fluoridation program.

These differences in spending patterns do not explain the U.S. health care cost problem, but they do suggest that there are significantly different ways in which countries can organize and finance health care services and suggest the key variables that should be examined to explain our cost problem. All of these developed countries, except Sweden with its abnormally high allocation to long-term care, allocate from 67 percent to nearly 80 percent of their health care spending for physicians, hospitals, and drugs. Consequently, our comparative analysis of national health care spending patterns will concentrate on these three expenditure groups and we should emphasize physician expenditures because the United States allocates significantly (over 30 percent) more of its health care spending to physicians.

Table 6.4 was also prepared from the Rublee-Schneider adjustment of the OECD data to show that the United States did not invest in more facilities or human resources devoted to health care compared to the six other countries. The United States does not have a larger supply of physicians for its population (fourth in the number of physi-

TABLE 6.4   Availability and Cost of Health Care Resources in Seven Developed Nations for 1988

Country	Phy. per 1,000	Cost per Phy.	Beds per 1,000	Cost Per Bed	Pharm. per 1,000	Cost Per Pharm.
Canada	2.2	$ 72,273	6.9	$105,072	0.80	$233,750
France	2.6	71,538	10.2	52,059	0.91	540,659
Germany	2.9	66,897	10.9	37,431	0.56	573,214
Japan	1.6	97,500	15.6	20,897	0.69	481,159
Sweden	2.9	47,241	13.3	46,842	0.51	370,588
U.K.	1.4	83,571	6.5	62,461	NA	NA
U.S.	2.3	182,174	5.1	170,196	0.66	275,758

Source: The cost per physician, per bed, and per pharmacist were based on the cost data from Rubles and Schneider [1991], and calculated with resource data from Schieber [1992].

cians per 1,000 population). It has the lowest quantity of hospital beds per 1,000, and the supply of pharmacists per capita is fourth. However, the U.S. cost per unit of physicians and hospital beds is substantially higher than any of the other countries. As was noted earlier, part of the reason that the cost per pharmacist is the fifth lowest of the six countries stems in part from the exclusion of hospital-administered drugs, which also has the effect of increasing the relative cost per hospital bed.

The U.S. cost per physician and per bed is much higher than the next highest nation's cost per unit of resource, almost 1.9 times the Japanese cost per physician and more than 1.6 times the Canadian cost per hospital bed, and these two components of health care costs constitute 64 percent of U.S. health care spending. The higher unit costs explain virtually all of the excess U.S. health care cost as measured by either the allocation of GDP or per capita health care costs. If, for example, the United States could have reduced its per physician and per bed cost to the level of the second most expensive nation in each of these two categories without increasing the supply of these resources or the utilization of resources in the other expense categories, the United States would have been able to lower its 1988 per capita health care cost from $2,006 to $1,472 and reduced it health care allocation of GDP from 11.1 to 8.4 percent, the fifth lowest allocation of the seven countries compared in 1988.

The practice patterns of doctors and hospitals and their consequent unit costs help us understand why the United States has such high health care costs. Because the unit cost per physician or per hospital bed is the product of the frequency of resource utilization, i.e., the number and kind of physician visits or the number and kind of hospital admissions and the charges for those services, these unit costs should be broken down into the quantity of resource utilization and the fees charged per unit of resource utilization. Unfortunately, the OECD data for the seven countries do not allow for a breakdown of physician or hospital unit costs in this manner. As a consequence, we shall use alternative data sources for the countries being compared.

We know, for example, that Japanese physicians in 1987 had 12.8 visits per capita versus 5.3 visits per capita in the United States and that Japanese surgeons performed 22 operations per 1,000 population in 1984 versus 91 operations per 1,000 population in the United

States in 1986 [Ikegami 1991]. These ratios suggest that Japanese physicians practice a much less intensive kind of medicine both inside and outside the hospital and charge much lower fees than their American counterparts. If the 1987 outpatient visit data were roughly comparable in 1988, the average cost of an outpatient visit in Japan was $12.19 versus $79.07 per visit in the United States. Japanese physicians had on average 8,000 patient visits per year while the average American physician had only 2,304 visits in 1988. That is, the cost per visit in the United States was roughly 6.5 times more than in Japan, but U.S. physicians partially made up for the higher cost by seeing only 29 percent as many patients as the average Japanese physician.

The Japanese physician's caseload is so prodigious because of a unique form of fee regulations that require all physicians, regard-of training or experience, to be paid the same charges for a particular procedure. Consequently, the only avenue available for Japanese physicians to increase their income is to see more patients, and all physicians without respect to specialty training provide primary or general care to obtain a sufficient patient volume. Ikegami [1991] concludes that "the uniform fee schedule has brought about both equity and cost containment" but it has also diluted the services provided. "In outpatient care, a clinic physician sees an average of forty-nine patients per day [with very short consultation times] and patients end up paying repeat visits to the clinics." There is little physician time for inpatient hospital care and, as we shall see, the Japanese operate their hospitals more like nursing homes.

However, there is room for U.S. physicians to increase patient visits without going to the extreme activity of the Japanese. For example, Fuchs and Hahn [1990] in a comparison of expenditures for physicians' services in the United States and Canada also found that the higher physician expenditures per capita in the United States "are explained almost entirely by higher fees; the quantity of physicians' services per capita is actually lower . . . [so that] despite the large disparity in fees, physicians' net incomes in the United States are only about one-third higher than in Canada." The U.S. ratio of physician income to the Japanese could be as much as 90 percent higher, depending on practice costs in the two countries.

The much higher level of physician fees in the United States is not simply a higher price for the same service, however. The U.S. physicians practice a style of medicine with much more high tech, specialist kind of care than the physians in just about any other developed nation, principally because of a much higher ratio of physician specialists to primary care physicians. Kosterlitz [1992b] has pointed out that in the United States, even with the supply of physicians growing 3.5 times faster than the population, "the percentage of physicians trained in primary care—already well below the 50 percent or more found in many other industrialized countries—has been falling steadily, and now stands at 32 percent." The economic consequences of this distribution of physicians is to lower physician productivity and increase health care costs, for, as Schroeder has noted, "Americans simply do not have enough health problems to keep all of our specialists appropriately occupied. Low rates of disease and a large capacity to treat it means many instances of too-aggressive care that produce only marginal improvements in health" [Kosterlitz 1992b].

The implications of the high tech, specialist style of care prevalent in the United States are also reflected in the way American hospitals are utilized. As the data in Table 6.4 indicated, the United States incurred an annual cost per hospital bed of $170,196, which was almost 62 percent higher than Canada, the second highest of the OECD nations in this comparison. Although the United States had the second lowest admission rate of the seven countries at 13.8 per 1,000 population in 1988 (Japan's rate was 7.8), it had the highest cost per admission of any country in the world of $6,290. Table 6.5 summarizes the cost and utilization data for the seven nations. It should be emphasized that, in order to maximize the amount of comparative information, the table is based on all hospitals, both long-term and short-term facilities, in the countries. The sixth or last column, which reports the percentage of acute patient days of the total patient days cared for in 1988, suggests that these national hospital systems are operated in two quite different ways. France, Japan (based on the very long length of stay), Sweden, and the U.K. operate hospital systems that actively utilize both long-term and short-term facilities; whereas Canada, Germany, and the United States, with 71, 66, and 69 percent acute to total patient days, respectively, basically operate short-term, acute hospital systems with long-term care being utilized in a secondary or ancillary role.

Of the three nations operating primarily in the acute care hospital mode, Germany operates most efficiently with lower costs per patient day and per stay, a lower staffing ratio per patient day, and a higher

TABLE 6.5   Hospital Cost and Utilization In Seven Developed Nations for 1988

Country*	Cost per Pat Day	Lgth of Stay*	Cost per Adm	Staff Ratio**	Occup %	Acute/ Tot Days***
Canada	$360	13.9	$5,000	2.40	84.9%	71%
France	192	13.1	2,518	1.04	81.2	50
Germany	118	16.1	1,898	1.27	86.5	66
Japan	80	52.1	4,179	.77	84.5	NA
Sweden	161	19.3	3,115	1.85	85.1	30
U.K.	170	15.0	2,553	2.60	80.6	45
U.S.	676	9.3	6,290	3.05	69.2	69

Source: Rublee and Schneider [1991] and Schieber et al [1992].

*(Average) Length of Stay
**Staffing Ratio (Full-Time Equivalents per Patient Day)
***Acute Patient Days (as a Percentage of) Total Patient Days

occupancy rate than Canada and the United States. Although Canada and the United States operate their hospital facilities in the same intense manner, the U.S. service costs substantially more. The per diem costs in the United States were nearly 88 percent higher than in Canada and its per stay costs were more than 25 percent higher, the smaller difference reflecting the shorter length of stay in the United States. Except for length of stay, the U.S. facilities have higher costs, higher staffing levels, and less efficient overall use of its hospital capacity than any of the other six nations.

One of the principal reasons for the higher hospital costs in the United States is the greater proliferation of major medical technologies in its hospitals, the so called "big ticket items." Table 6.6 compares the number of six major kinds of technologies per million people in these three countries. The United States in 1987 had significantly more of each of the six technology units per million people, varying from a low of only 21 percent more organ transplant units than Canada to a high of 292 percent in magnetic resonance imaging (MRI) units. Even though the United States has a poorer record of utilizing its hospital facilities than the other two countries, the availability of such a larger number of these six major technologies translates into the delivery of more open heart surgeries, more cardiac catheterizations, more organ transplants, more radiation therapy, more lithotripsic

TABLE 6.6   Availability of Selected Technologies in Canada, Germany, and United States for 1987

Technology Units Per Million	Canada	Germany	U.S.	U.S. Ratio to Second Most*
Open-heart surgeries	1.23	.74	3.26	2.65
Cardiac catheterization	1.50	2.64	5.06	1.92
Organ transplantation	1.08	.46	1.31	1.21
Radiation therapy	.54	3.13	3.97	1.26
Lithotripsy	.16	.34	.94	2.76
Magnetic resonance imaging	.46	.94	3.69	3.92

Source: Rublee [1989] with 1987 data for Germany and the United States and 1989 data for Canada.

*(Number of units in) U.S. Ratio (to number of units in the country with) Second Most (units)

operations, and more imaging in the United States than in Canada and Germany.

Thus, the primary reason for the higher hospital costs in the United States is precisely the same reason that the U.S. physician costs are so much higher—hospital and doctor services in the United States have adopted an extremely intense, high tech, specialized style of care. The overinvestment in health care reflects the choice of technology that the United States has made and the comprehensiveness with which that technology choice has been applied. Other countries have chosen much less capital-intensive care technologies that utilize fewer resources in aggregate, even though the United States does not have more doctors and hospital beds per capita than the other countries.

The Fundamental Difference: U.S. Style of Medicine

The difference in resource utilization between the high tech, specialized style of medicine practiced in the United States and the low tech, primary style of care given in many of these other developed nations was well illustrated by Professor Howard H. Hiatt [1992]. Hiatt contrasted the treatment of two cases in the United Kingdom and the United States, a patient in his mid-80s suffering from severe heart disease who develops rectal bleeding and a 13-month old child of a teenage mother who develops acute bronchitis. Neither patient would be treated in a hospital in the United Kingdom because the patients' general practitioner (GP), who makes house calls, could diagnose and prescribe the appropriate therapy without any additional resources. Although the elderly patient probably has cancer of the bowel, his GP knows that confirmation of this diagnosis will not affect the eventual outcome of the case. Hospitalization will only cause substantial discomfort to his patient who prefers to receive care in the comfort of his home from the GP and a visiting nurse. In the United States the patient's cardiologist would most likely hospitalize the man and subject him to a battery of very unpleasant tests that would only confirm the cancer diagnosis, but not alter the appropriate therapy. The additional resource cost in the United States would be several thousand dollars.

Similarly, the infant in the United Kingdom would receive a prescription for an antibiotic after the GP's house call and administration of the initial dose of the medicine. The young mother would also receive assistance in obtaining other social services as well as follow-up visits for her baby. In the United States the young mother would have to take public transportation to the nearest hospital emergency room to obtain care for her baby. After hours of waiting, she would probably receive the same antibiotic, but at substantially higher cost to the state's Medicaid program because of the ER visit and the number of laboratory tests and X-rays required for diagnosis. The additional net cost in the United States would be several hundred dollars for more scientific and technological medicine than in the United Kingdom.

Hiatt's hypothetical cases illustrate the so called "little ticket" technologies that are more pervasive in the practice of medicine in the United States than the major, "big ticket" technologies discussed earlier in the comparative review of hospital facilities. Little ticket high-tech health care, e.g., all of the clinical lab tests and noncomputerized x-rays, simply because of the much higher frequency of use in the U.S. health care system, are more insidious to the American style of medicine than the big ticket items. Moloney and Rogers even advanced the thesis in 1979 that "the few big, highly visible technologies such as the CT scanner actually account for far less of the annual growth in medical expenditures than do the collective expense of thousands of small tests and procedures that are more frequently used by physicians and that individually cost very little." The implications of this thesis for health care cost containment in the United States are very troubling because the thesis implies that the high-tech approach is embedded in the fabric of the practice style of U.S. medicine.

WHY DID AMERICANS OVERINVEST IN SCIENTIFIC MEDICINE?

The international comparsions have shown that Americans have developed a more high-tech, specialized style of health care practice than any other developed nation in the world. They also pinpoint the exact time when the U.S. investment became excessive. The implementation of the Medicare program on July 1, 1966, and Medicaid on January 1, 1967, were the key dates after which Americans began outspending the rest of the world on health care. These two huge federal programs, without adequate controls, pumped so many resources into the U.S. health care system that it exaggerated the system's existing predisposition for a scientific and technological style of medicine.

However, in order to understand what key market relationships were stretched by Medicare and Medicaid it will be helpful to reconsider the historical development of the U.S. health care system as described in the previous chapters. The factors that exaggerated the role of high health care technology and specialization in the post-1965 period need to be identified and contrasted with the restraints on the growth of technology and specialization in other developed nations.

The Development of the U.S. Health Care Market

The U.S. bias for science and technology began at the turn of the century. Advocates of scientific medicine colluded to gain control of the American Medical Association as a means of reforming American medical education to train future physicians according to the tenets of scientific medicine, a school of medicine that had been imported to the United States from Europe. In addition, they conspired to control medical staff appointments in most large urban and all teaching hospitals in order to restrict the more invasive practice of medicine to those trained or qualified in scientific medicine. These arrangements separated the market for health care services in urban areas into primary/generalist care and specialist/technologist care.

That separation in the Great Depression led to a revolt by the AMA, whose principal GP members had become greatly disadvantaged economically, against the development of competitive forms of health insurance that could have contributed to the development of integrated, comprehensive health care delivery and financing organizations. Instead, Blue Cross and Blue Shield were founded in the '30s to preserve the free choice of physicians and a fee-for-service payment arrangement that did not include out-of-hospital insurance benefits. Even though commercial insurers subsequently came to "compete" with the Blues for the marketing of health insurance, there were no significant changes in the organization of the health care market for the next 50 years.

Some totally unrelated events unfolded during and after World War II that greatly expanded the financing of health care services. Between April 1943, with President Roosevelt's executive order granting wage control authority to the War Labor Board, and June 23, 1947, when Congress passed the Labor Management Relations Act (the Taft-Hartley Act) by overriding President Truman's veto, a series of unrelated and largely unplanned actions were taken by a host of federal government agencies that encouraged the basic American predisposition for a high-tech, specialized health care style and established sources of funds for financing that style of care. The following events were the catalysts for the subsequent development of the American health care financing and delivery system:

* The War Labor Board's ruling that fringe benefits (including health insurance) were exempt from the mandatory wage controls

* Passage of the Public Service Act of 1944, which included the authority to award research grants to nonfederal entities

* The Veterans Administration ruling that payment of tuition and living allowances could be made to hospitals and to physicians taking graduate training in acceptable hospitals under the Serviceman's Readjustment Act of 1944, "the GI Bill"

* Passage of the Hospital Survey and Construction Act of 1946, "the Hill-Burton Act," which provided federal grants for financing hospital construction, especially in rural communities

* Passage of the Labor Management Relations Act, "Taft-Hartley," which included a provision requiring trust fund control of employer contributions for employee welfare.

These five actions of the federal government, coupled with continued popular support, created the environment in which scientific medicine thrived.

As was discussed in chapter 3, labor unions led the way in obtaining health insurance benefits for the employed as a result of the agency rulings and Taft-Hartley provisions. The National Institutes of Health administered a billion dollars in research grants to health scientists and institutions in the next 20 years. Later, federal support for medical and health professions education and construction of research facilities was added. Physician education and encouragement of specialization was financed through the GI Bill, which carried on the medical specialist norm that had been observed in military care during the war. In addition, hospital facilities suited to specialist care were made available across the entire nation.

Ironically, the AMA built its reputation as a powerful political force in America by obstructionist tactics that were harmful to its principal constituents, general practitioners. Its opposition to health insurance in the 1930s and Medicare in the 1950s and 60s caused health insurance benefits to encourage a high-tech, specialized style of medicine practiced in hospitals rather than the high-touch, caring style of primary care practiced by generalists and family physicians. In addition, the AMA's opposition in the post-World War II period to federal government support for medical education resulted in strengthening academic or specialist medicine, again at the expense of primary care physicians.

The direction and emphasis for the U.S. health care system had been established, and, because of the political popularity of these programs, subsequent federal actions continued to support high-tech and specialized health care, even if few understood it. When shortages of primary care physicians developed in the '60s and '70s, larger federal grant programs were approved to support the education of more physicians, even though the newly educated physicians chose specialization in even larger numbers. When the physician specialists needed more support personnel, Congress and the Administration obliged with health manpower training funds for the education of nurses and medical technicians. When retirees, who had become accustomed to the benefits of the American health care system but were no longer eligible for employer-purchased health insurance, became dissatisfied, Medicare was fashioned and approved to resemble as closely as possible those employer-sponsored private health insurance plans. In fact, the program would be administered through the same private health insurance carriers, and the preamble to the legislation promised that the federal government would not interfere in the practice of medicine.

When the Medicare-Medicaid programs were implemented, the U.S. health insurance market reached the saturation point for "free" first or low dollar coverage and disenfranchised the consumer as a determining force in the health care market. These government programs had been constructed to emulate the politically popular private health insurance plans without recognizing that private health insurance had, "For all practical purposes . . . no controls on the providers. Hospitals were paid cost or charges, whichever was lower; physicians were paid their usual and customary fees" [Anderson 1985, 263].

The goal of all federal health programs approved after World War II, despite the lack of an overall plan of development, became the emulation of what had worked previously in the private sector's development of the nation's health care system. However, this approach was taken not just to accommodate doctors and hospitals, but, more important, to accommodate the wishes of the American people, who were thrilled by the accomplishments of modern medical science and were proud of their local hospitals. In spite of the higher health care costs that such a system generated, the health care system is still very popular with the American people, much more popular than the frugal Japanese health care system is with the Japanese people.

These federal goverment programs ensured the central role of scientific medicine in the development and operation of the U.S. health care system. However, accommodation, beginning with organized medicine's acceptance of the Flexner Report's recommendations for restructuring medical education prior to America's entry into World War I in exchange for the grandfathering of unscientifically trained and unqualified physicians, has been the means for assimilating scientific medicine into this nation's health care system. In the 1920s surgeons and scientifically-trained physicians captured control of the medical staff appointments in the better urban and medical-school-affiliated hospitals by reaching accommodation with hospital management over the apportionment of patient revenues. In the 1930s these same hospitals and physician groups provided the leadership for an accommodation with Blue Cross in the development of voluntary private health insurance. However, the accommodations that were reached in the 1940s, first with employers over the purchase of private health insurance and then with the federal government to institution-alize the insurance benefits relationship and to subsidize health care research, education, and facilities, were the capstones for the control of the U.S. health care industry's subsequent development by advo-cates of scientific medicine.

This series of accommodations reflected incremental responses to changes in the socioeconomic environment, often subtly influenced by the dynamic leadership and promoters of scientific medicine. That portion of the medical community certainly had been much more influential than advocates of community or preventive medicine. Even the addition of a publicly-funded health insurance program for the aged represented an incremental approach to national health insur-ance. However, its implementation proved to be the proverbial straw that broke the camel's back.

After the implementation of the Medicare-Medicaid programs the allocation of U.S. resources to health care became almost one-third higher than the allocations made by other developed nations. The U.S. share of its GDP allocated to health care more than doubled while the six other nations increased their allocations by just over 150 percent. Two quite different kinds of inflation occurred. The programs were initially followed by a huge increase in health care costs, the so-called Medicare cost bulge, and continued the existing pattern of health care spending; i.e., the largest increase in costs occurred with hospitals (see chapter 4). This was the last gasp of the original strain of health care inflation that had grown out of the early noncompete agreements between hospitals and doctors. It was also a continuation, at a higher rate, of the demand-pull inflation produced through the growth in health insurance coverage.

Eventually the proportion of health care dollars spent for hospital services began to fall and the proportion spent for physician services began to rise. There was no comparable increase in health insurance coverage for any population segment accompanying the second spurt of health care inflation, but there had been a gradual and cumulative expansion in the coverage for outpatient benefits. In addition, the Medicare program accorded full payment status to ambulatory surgi-centers in 1983. Meanwhile, the number of physician specialists had been growing so rapidly that there was mounting pressure on physicians to increase the number of services provided per patient contact as well as the number of outpatient surgical procedures. Thus, the second growth phase might more aptly be described as a supplier-induced expansion. Doctors were no longer inhibited by the lack of ambulatory insurance coverage or their decades-old noncompete agreement with hospitals. It was not simply an extension of the demand-pull, growth of health insurance coverage, kind of health care cost inflation.

What Made It Cost So Much?

Despite the U.S. health care system's popularity for scientific achievement and therapeutic advances, it costs too much. Why? The simple answer is that in reaching these incremental accommodations the cost restraints necessary for the operation of a cost-effective health care delivery system were diminished or eliminated. This lack of restraints can be seen by considering the experiences of the other six developed nations cited earlier in this chapter. Although all six nations were operated through publicly financed health care systems, that model need not be adopted to allocate resources more prudently to health care providers. It is, however, a model that should be considered in the debate over health care reform.

The objective is to identify those restraints on the allocation of resources these six nations have that the United States is missing. In all six countries a centralized budget determines how much of the nation's resources will be devoted to health care, and there is a system for allocating these resources to specific programs for the care of people. Health care providers periodically appeal to the legislatures for additional funds for improved care, and, after the budget allotment has been determined, they appeal to the public servants in the government as to how best to spend that allotment. If additional funds are allocated to health care beyond the available government revenues, taxes must be raised to finance the larger expenditures. This political tension regulates the quantity of resources allocated to health care. This system has the merit of disclosing alternatives and their consequences. In the final analysis the electorate expresses its satisfaction with these allocative decisions by periodically reviewing the records of the elected representatives. In this review process, however, health care is just one of many important issues on which the electorate must base its judgment. If, for example, the Japanese could vote directly on their satisfaction with their health care system, it is likely that additional resources would be allocated to improving their system. Americans have generally preferred a system in which preferences can be expressed in the marketplace, where people vote with dollars on what they wish to purchase and how much they are willing to pay for a particular good or service. The marketplace usually creates sufficient tension between buyers and sellers to make it an efficient allocator of resources, i.e., the resulting allocation is a very close approximation of what most people want. Such market tension has decreased in the American health care marketplace since World War II. The problem became especially acute in the late 1970s and 1980s when many employers tried to apply market controls by raising premium contributions and increasing copayments and deductibles in their employees' benefits, but there was no appreciable reduction in the rate of health care cost increases. The reason for this lack of marketplace response to the increased employee costs of health care appears to be that the changes have not kept up with the rate of aggregate health care cost increases because the average level of consumer spending as a percentage of disposable income has not increased (see chapter 5). It has increased as a percent of personal (before taxes) income only because of the continual increase in the Medicare payroll tax.

For most American consumers there is no binding budget constraint on health care expenditures. That, coupled with private insurers' and government's failure to impose any effective cost controls on providers, has created a tensionless void in the health care marketplace. Physicians, primarily specialists who were the direct descendants of the early advocates of scientific medicine, stepped into that void and, almost by default, came to dominate the health care market. The U.S. health care market has lost its anchor and thus its capacity to apply tension to the consumer choice of health care services because of the growth of first or low-dollar health insurance. In the post-World War II marketplace, consumer spending for health care remained at less than 5 percent of the consumer's disposable income as total health spending came to constitute more than 14 percent of total consumption expenditures in the United States. The public and private health insurance programs have financed all of the increased expenditures for health care in the United States since 1940.

The expansion of the health care industry was virtually painless for the average consumer. Only recently concern bordering on paranoia about the health insurance implications of loss of employment brought the health care cost issue to the consumer's attention. Because of the prevalence of first or low-dollar health insurance, consumers behave as if what they pay directly for services is the cost of care, even though it is only a small portion of the total cost. Why not see a specialist instead of a GP when the cost differential is so small for the consumer.

Furthermore, the health insurance policy provided by the consumer's employer had become "free" to the majority of consumers. Most current employees have never had to choose between cash wages and health insurance coverage. Employees have learned since entering the workplace that employer-purchased health insurance is a good deal because no income taxes are imposed on that benefit. More employees have become aware of the cash value of the benefit as the two-worker family has emerged and only one of the two employers provides insurance, but most employees have continued to ignore the effect of insurance on cash wages even with larger copayments, deductibles, and premium payments.

Unintended Consequences

In effect, the consumer through the acceptance of employer-purchased health insurance has abdicated the usual role in the marketplace of determining the kind and quantity of health care services that the consumer wishes to purchase. In the U.S. health care marketplace those decisions have been made largely by those physicians, generally advocates of scientific medicine, who prefer high-tech, specialized care over high-touch, primary care.

More than 50 years ago J. M. Clark defined competitive controls as "a system of mutual compulsion which forces everyone in a business to do what no one of them would choose to do if competition did not compel him . . . . If competition did not exercise this kind of coercion, it would never reduce prices, weed out inefficient producers, and apply the spur of ruthless necessity to the others, all for the benefit of the public" [Clark 1939, 136]. In the health insurance market that developed in the United States, there was no mutual compulsion among physicians to inhibit the overspecialization of physician resources or to encourage their participation in comprehensive health care delivery organizations.

In the late 1970s and 1980s, when the full effect of the Medicare program's expansion of health insurance coverage had been absorbed, the lack of the U.S. health care marketplace's responsiveness to consumer wants or needs became especially evident by the increasing number of new physicians choosing specialties over primary care. These new physicians were able to select their specialty based on their own wants without any concern about the economic consequences that would normally be reflected in lowering future incomes as the number of specialists rose. In other words, as the consumers failed to incur appreciably higher costs in seeing specialists rather than GPs, the labor market for physicians also ceased to reflect the relative treatment value of different specialties to consumer wants. In order to operate effectively the health care market must have consumers that respond to alternatives based on the total magnitude of cost differentials, not just the consumer's out-of-pocket costs.

The final step for physician dominance of the health care market was achieved early in the 1980s without much concerted action by physicians. Both public and private health insurers redesigned their benefit structures to reduce the longstanding bias favoring the hospital site for insurance coverage. The rationale for parity in coverage was the argument that out-of-hospital services were much more economical than in-hospital services, which is correct as far as unit costs are concerned.

Thus by 1980 physicians were drawn into a position in the health care marketplace where they could do almost whatever they wished without fear of significant economic consequences—most consumers didn't care due to the absence of a budget constraint on their health care spending. Physicians were encouraged to move their services out of the hospital, whose peer review controls could be much more stringent than an insurance company's bureaucratic review process that was preoccupied with maximizing discounts on fictitious prices.

A market dominanted by any supplier group will soon reflect that group's wants and desires, not the consumer's. So it was in the health care industry in the 1980s and '90s. Physicians entering the health care market chose to specialize in increasing numbers because they preferred problem solving and technology over direct patient care and because they could specialize without sacrificing future earnings. Normally a labor market will work to reduce the earnings of categories of workers that are in excess supply, but the health care market has not imposed such penalties on the over-supply of physician specialists, whose incomes continue to be substantially higher than those of primary care physicians.

In addition, there were even greater rewards for those physicians who chose both to specialize and to establish or invest in their own out-of-hospital ambulatory care enterprises. Even with lower unit costs, the effect of the unbundling of hospital services into enterprises owned or controlled by physician entrepreneurs has been to increase total health care costs because the increase in the quantity of services provided has been greater than the reduction in unit costs. The substantial increase in the numbers of high-tech facilities and services outside the hospital in this period reflects the profitability of this business strategy.

Even before the latest round of excesses in the health care market Dr. John Freymann summarized the effects of the scientific medicine movement as follows:

What they [the early 20th century advocates of scientific medicine] did merits admiration, but in solving the problems of their own times they created others for ours. Their magnificent achievements and the unintended consequences of their actions epitomize the curse that threads through the history of health care: imbalance. We have gone from no science to little but science, from no specialists to practically all specialists, from widespread fear of hospitals to widespread idolization of them, from insufficient funding to financing that overloaded the system, from worship of research *qua* research to disenchantment with basic investigation and demand for "practical" results, from life that lived with death to a lifespan that is almost guaranteed, from lavish support of one fragment of the system to neglect of the other three [preventive, mental health, and long term care], from an adundance of almost uniformly inadequate doctors to a maldistributed and insufficient number of almost uniformly good ones, from the over-confidence of ignorance to the paralysis of more knowledge than anyone can encompass, from inadequate vocational training by disinterested pracitioners to irrelevant scientific education by disinterested researchers [Freymann 1974, 96].

What the '80s and '90s have added to Freymann's list of imbalances in health care is the movement *from a market in which the consumer was king to one in which the physician is king*. Even though this change may also have been an unintended consequence, health care reform must redress this role reversal because price competition and market controls can only be effective in consumer-dominated markets. The political difficulty in restoring consumers to their proper market role is getting those consumers who are able to accept some financial responsibility for their health care spending.

THE PRINCIPAL SOURCE OF MARKET FAILURE

This study of more than 90 years of U.S. health care market experience places the blame for uncontrolled health care costs squarely on the failure of the health insurance mechanism to develop beyond the "free choice of physician" model that was created by compromise between hospitals and GPs during the 1930s. Of the anticompetitive agreements that were entered into in the pre-World War II market, only the primacy of "free choice" model of health insurance has survived subsequent market developments.

Altough the "free choice" model was initially supported by the misguided and sometimes illegal efforts of the American Medical Association to assist GPs in maintaining independence from the hospital practice model in their competition with specialists, various wartime and postwar developments in the U.S. labor market eventually became the model's sustaining force. First or low-dollar health insurance "freely" provided by employers became the norm in America, outlasting motherhood, apple pie, and Chevrolet as the American icon. When the federal government made that insurance model an entitlement for all elderly Americans, its inherent weakness as a device for providing sufficient tension in the marketplace to control health care costs became apparent.

It is important to understand that the reason "free choice" first-dollar health insurance caused such disastrous cost containment results is that it has diminished the consumer's sensitivity to the real cost consequences of health care consumption decisions. It is clear that in decisions about specific health services, like visiting a doctor, having surgery, or filling a prescription, the relevant consumer cost becomes the out-of-pocket service charge. However, for aggregate choices, like the kind of health insurance or managed care organization membership to have the employer purchase on the consumer's behalf, the relevant cost is more the employee's share of the premium. It must also include the net out-of-pocket expenditures that the consumer expects to have to make over the term of the insurance policy or period of membership in the HMO. If the managed care organization or HMO places a high out-of-pocket cost on purchasing physician services outside the organization, consumers place a high priority on wanting to buy physician services outside the managed care organization. This preference is evidenced by their reluctance to join a staff or closed panel HMO and the popularity of including a fixed and only nominally higher copayment provision for out-of-plan physician services.

The dominant employer-provided "free choice" low or first-dollar insurance coverage has distorted the consumer's view of health costs both on the purchase of specific health care services and on the aggregate choice of kind of health insurance or health plan. The costs to the consumer are always understated on specific services, and the savings that accrue to the consumer from joining a more restricted choice and lower cost health plan are less than the overall cost savings that the plan can generate in total. In other words, why should an employee save money for an employer? Consumers continue to prefer fewer restrictions on their purchases of health services than they would have been willing to accept if "free" first-dollar coverage with freedom of choice of physician had not become the market norm by which all other plans would be judged. In addition, the working consumer's bias for higher, less restrictive coverage is further encouraged by U.S. tax policies that permit the employee to avoid paying income taxes on the employer's health insurance contribution even though these benefits are clearly a vital part of the employee's compensation.

However, persons 65 and over, who have been given entitlement to a low-dollar "free choice of physician" health insurance policy, have even less incentive than those under 65 to join a restrictive, but more cost effective health plan. In many respects the Medicare program's lack of consumer cost containment incentives is more serious than the problems with employee health insurance plans because the aged are much more intensively in need of health services. Not only was this group the fastest growing age segment in the U.S. population, going from 9.5 percent in 1965 to 12.2 percent of all Americans in 1987, but the use of health care services and, especially, inpatient hospital services, by the aged increased even more rapidly. In 1965, the United States spent 23.8 percent of total personal health expenditures on persons 65 and over, by 1977 30 percent of the spending was devoted to aged persons, and by 1987 36.3 percent of the

TABLE 6.7   Health Care Spending by Age Distribution of U.S. Population in 1965, 1977, and 1987

Age Groups	1965 % of Pop.	1965 % of Spdg.	1977 % of Pop.	1977 % of Spdg.	1987 % of Pop.	1987 % of Spdg.
Under 19	38.9%	17.1%	31.9%	13.0%	27.6%	11.6%
19 to 64	51.6	59.1	57.3	57.0	60.3	52.1
65 and over	9.5	23.8	10.8	30.0	12.2	36.3
Total	100.0%	100.0%	100.0%	100.0%	100.1%	100.0%

Source: The 1965 data are from Fisher [1980] and the 1977 and 1987 data are from Waldo et al [1989].

total was consumed by the elderly [Fisher 1980, and Waldo et al 1989]. Table 6.7 reports the percentage of population and health care spending for all three age groups: those under 19, those 19 to 64, and those 65 and over. Although the United States is spending an increasing portion of its personal health care dollar on aged persons, the primary reason for this increased allocation to the aged persons is simply the increased percentage of aged persons in the overall population of the United States. During the initial 12 years when the Medicare program had its most pronounced demand-pull effects, from 1965 to 1977, per capita spending on the aged increased from $472 to $1,856 or 293 percent, which was a much higher rate of increase than for children or nonaged adults during this period. However, in the decade from 1977 to 1987 the aged per capita health care spending grew more slowly than the other age groups. One of the reasons that spending on the aged relative to the rest of the population rose less rapidly in the latter period was the success of the federal government's oligopsonist purchasing practices in shifting their costs to the private insurer for the under-65 year olds; as Chapter 5 indicates the aged's relative share of hospital utilization, for example, continued to increase. In any event, over the entire 22 years, there was very little change in the relative allocation of personal health care resources among the three age groups, but the aged will continue to be the fastest growing age group in the United States for the foreseeable future.

The point is that consumers of all ages must become more cost conscious through the better design of health insurance benefits for both the employed and the entitled if the existing failure is to be corrected in the health care market. Health care reform without significant changes in the Medicare program's health insurance benefits is doomed to failure. As was cited earlier, the Rand study found that health care costs were nearly one-third less for persons with relatively large deductibles or, at least, 25 percent coinsurance provisions than for those individuals having free care (first-dollar coverage), and without any observable effect on health except for lower income families [Brooks, et al., 1983].

In addition, the problem with health insurance in the United States stems not only from the illusion of lower health care costs for consumers. In the private insurance market there are perverse incentives that encourage unacceptable behavior by insurance companies seeking to avoid writing insurance for those high risk persons who most need health insurance. The perverse incentive problem arises because of first-dollar coverage and the fact that illnesses and accidents are not randomly distributed across the population. An understanding of the private health insurance market must begin with the Roos et al [1989] findings that over a 16-year period about 50 percent of the population had few, other than routine, health care needs over their lifetimes; 45 percent incurred substantial lifetime health care costs; and the remaining 5 percent had extraordinary health care problems and expenses over their lives. Obviously, insurers would like to insure the healthy half of the population and, even more important, avoid the unhealthy 5 percent, which has led to discriminatory insurance and employment practices. Health care reform must also fix this problem.

In the next and last chapter the Clinton health reform proposal will be examined in terms of its capability to correct the deficiencies in the health care market that have been identified through this historical examination of the health care industry. That is, an evaluation will be made of its potential for making consumers and insurers sufficiently responsible to restore the effectiveness of the health care marketplace.

7

The Promise of Health Care Reform

The time has come to test the underlying premise of this study—that understanding the historical economic development of the health care industry can be helpful in constructing an effective proposal for reforming the health care market. A corollary of that premise, which in many respects may be easier to prove, is that the study of the history of health care reform itself is useful in evaluating current reform proposals. Although the histories of health care and its proposed reform may both affirm the biblical proverb that there is nothing new under the sun, the health care industry is still evolving; and its development has been so sensitive to unpredictable changes in knowledge and technology that it seems to defy those historical limitations.

The number of ways in which health care can be reformed, on the other hand, seems to be more limited because all reform proposals must answer some specific political and economic questions. Although the objectives for reform have changed over the nearly eight decades under consideration, the fundamental issues of what benefits are to be provided, to whom, by what system of health care delivery, and who is going pay for those benefits have been immutable. The continuing difficulty has been to obtain a large enough consensus on these issues to enact national health insurance (NHI) legislation. Indeed, part of our difficulty in obtaining agreement has been a deep-seated concern that any NHI system will restrain those unpredictable advances in scientific knowledge and technology that are the hallmark of the U.S. health care industry.

However, in the 1990s America seems ready at last to enact NHI legislation because of the extending duration of constantly rising health care costs. Americans can no longer afford to postpone the enactment of NHI. The current opportunity costs in terms of other social and educational programs that must be forgone as well as the overall health of our economy are too great for further delay.

Consequently, it is time to assess the options available for resolving our NHI questions and to implement NHI programs. Clearly, the front runner among those options is President Clinton's reform proposal, which will serve as the springboard for the consideration of NHI legislative proposals. After conducting that review in terms of the historical perspective that has served as the framework for this study, a compromise proposal will be presented that meets most of the general criteria for NHI plus the unique one that has been established in the historical analysis of the health care marketplace. Needless to say, that compromise proposal is not new, but much like President Clinton's is an amalgamation of old ideas in a new context reflecting current priorities.

THE CLINTON REFORM PROPOSAL

First of all, it is important to understand that President Clinton's leadership and concurrence is necessary for the passage of health care reform legislation. Some of the president's contributions have been unequivocally positive in moving the nation toward a consensus. Others can only be classified as ambiguous, both in terms of the process being incomplete and of necessary trade-offs in which the costs may exceed the benefits.

President Clinton recognized during the 1992 presidential campaign that health care reform was of major concern to the electorate. His decision to make health care reform his highest domestic priority next to job creation was significant. Because of the legislative calendar, he had to give priority to the 1993–94 federal budget and deficit reduction, and then the ratification of the North American Free Trade Agreement. Despite these delays and a prolonged bill drafting process, the Clinton administration was extremely successful in maintaining public interest and generating continuing support for health care reform even though the reform issue's priority has fallen slightly in the national public opinion polls. The Clinton plan has responded to shifting public opinion by combining the health security objective in the reform proposal with job and personal security goals to make overall security the overarching goal of his legislative program.

As a result of these efforts health care has received so much attention in the news media that an excellent public education program has been disseminated broadly—a necessary step for the enactment of any NHI legislation. The Clinton administration deserves much credit for orchestrating an effective public information campaign for its health care reform proposal through Hillary Rodham Clinton's involvement in the drafting task force and the initial congressional presentations, all of which have piqued the public's interest in health care reform.

By word and deed the president has established his understanding and commitment to the proposition that controlling health care costs is vital to the broader U.S. interests of converting consumption expenditures into solving the nation's budget deficit problems and making new social investments. So long as government is bound to its obligation to pay a proportional share of the ever rising health care bill, adequate funds can never be available for necessary debt reduction, improved education programs, or reinvestment in the nation's infrastructure.

On the other hand, the president's health care reform strategy has produced a must-win situation. The result is a reform plan that is flawed. First, the proposal has been drafted to avoid or minimize several politically sensitive issues, such as the plan's financing without imposing any controversial new taxes and preserving all the existing Medicare benefits. Second, the proposal has been drafted in a less than forthright manner. For example, it is dressed in market reform garb when in fact it represents a regulatory approach to containing health care costs through price or premium controls. Third, as a result of this overriding political pragmatism and the need for misdirection in the legislation, it is the longest and most complex NHI proposal ever drafted. It will challenge the congressional committee review process due to the number of committees that can claim jurisdiction over various parts of the proposal.

However, because of its comprehensiveness and universality of benefits, the proposal has the potential for passage and, with revision, can (1) cope adequately with the existing flaws in the health care marketplace, (2) enhance permanent job opportunities by amending the content of labor-management bargaining negotiations, and (3) reform the nature of federal entitlements for the middle and upper-income groups.

Because of the overallocation of resources to health care, the significance of health benefits in wage negotiations, and the misdirection of federal budget dollars in existing health care programs, the objectives for health care reform must extend beyond providing universal access to health care and restoring effectiveness in the health care marketplace. The problems in the health care market are the product of both systemic market and political failures. Consideration and passage of health reform legislation presents the most propitious time to confront the totality of our past failures. It is not a time to allow political sensitivities to perpetuate those errors by our unwillingness to face difficult political issues.

The tactical weakness of the Clinton proposal by conceding too soon on many of the most vital issues of health care reform can be offset by another tactic that the president has adopted. From the plan's unveiling, the president and all his spokespersons have professed no pride of authorship and a willingness to compromise on any of the provisions in the legislation as long as the Congress passes a bill in which "Every American and legally resident alien would have a personal health care card [that serves] as a promise that insurance would never be cancelled, even for people who fall ill or lose their jobs " [Clymer 1993]. The president's very specific bottom line for the legislation together with a broad proposal before the Congress provides an excellent framework for the debate on health care reform, and his determination to pass such legislation has given that debate the necessary urgency for action.

A Summary of the Clinton Plan

The Clinton NHI plan, unveiled in the fall of 1993, was generally or, at least, nominally consistent with his campaign rhetoric. It called for managed competition of the health care delivery system and for financing primarily through mandated coverage at place of employment with employers required to pay 80 percent of the premiums of the weighted-regional-average cost of the basic benefits. Subsidies were provided for small businesses, and the federal government assumed the employer responsibility for persons who had taken early retirement and were not yet eligible for Medicare.

Clinton's program would be administered through state governments, but coordination and direction would come from a National Health Board, consisting of seven members appointed by the president with the advice and consent of the Senate, that would set national standards and oversee the state program administration. The states would establish state plans designating an agency to administer subsidies for low-income individuals or families and employers, to certify health plans (the delivery organization and/or insurer), to regulate the finances of the health plans, administer data collection and quality management and improvement programs, and establish the geographic area and governance of Regional Health Alliances. The alliances are responsible for representing the interests of consumers and purchasers of health care services, structuring the market for health care services, and ensuring that all residents in an area who are covered through the regional alliance enroll in health plans that provide the nationally guaranteed benefits.

The health plans, which have been certified by the responsible state agency, provide the coverage of these benefits by contracting with either the regional alliances or directly with larger corporate employers. The plans may offer the NHI benefits on the traditional fee-for-service basis, a capitated HMO benefit that meets or exceeds the national benefit, and a combination fee-for-service and capitation approach. Both HMO registrants and subscribers to the combination approach must have the ability, at a fixed additional fee, to purchase services outside the plan's physicians or facilities. This alternative and an expansion in the number of fee-for-service plans allowed were added to the legislative proposal after a number of objections were raised about the reduced freedom of choice of physicians in the original draft of the proposal.

The rates approved by the regional alliances for fee-for-service insurance, combination plans, and capitated HMOs would be calculated on a community-wide basis, not on an experience rating system. However, corporate purchasers would have greater latitude. Provider charges in fee-for-service plans would be established by the regional alliance, which could operate on an established fee schedule and/or require prospective budgeting approval of the fee-for-service providers.

The mandated health insurance benefits were quite comprehensive, better than the current Medicare benefits and, at least, equivalent to all but the best of current employer-provided coverage. The benefits included hospital and emergency services; the services of physicians and other health professionals; home health care, hospice, and extended-care services; outpatient laboratory, diagnostic, and rehabilitation services; outpatient drugs; some preventive dental care for children; durable medical equipment and devices; vision and hearing care; and some health education classes. The only significant controversies about the benefits package concerned abortion services, which are included; the frequency of mammograms, which was increased; and the lack of parity in benefits between mental and physical illness because Clinton followed the current insurance practice of qualifying or limiting mental health benefits. Three types of cost sharing plans must be offered with these benefits; a low, a high, and a combination cost sharing plans. However, the high cost sharing plan has a modest annual deductible of $200 per individual and $400 per family, coinsurance of 20 percent, and a limit of $1,500 per individual and $3,000 per family.

This is a very brief summary of a 1,342-page legislative proposal of extreme complexity. More details will be presented as it is analyzed in relationship to two other NHI proposals. One is the "Jackson Hole Group" proposal for *The 21st Century American Health System, A Proposal for Reform*, which was generally believed to be the prototype for much of the structure and organization of the Clinton plan.[22] The other is the original Health Security Act, which was introduced by Senator Edward M. Kennedy of Massachusetts in August 1970 and offered "cradle to grave" health insurance coverage to all Americans through federal financing and regulation of the health care delivery system.

A Wolf in Sheep's Clothing

Both the ideas of the Jackson Hole Group and their terminology in President Clinton's September 22, 1993, speech to the Congress introducing the American Health Security Act and in the language of the bill itself suggested to many that "the Clinton plan aims to achieve these goals by *restructuring the health care market to foster competition on price and quality*, building on the employer-provided insurance base to cover all Americans" [White, 1993, emphasis added]. However, if the Jackson Hole Group's proposal is managed care, then Clinton's plan has a more direct linkage to Kennedy's 1970 formulation and may be more appropriately described as regulated-provider competition.

The managed competition idea sought to encourage consumers to enroll in integrated health care delivery and financing organizations by getting "Employer and government sponsors . . . to convert to defined-contribution health benefits programs, limit tax-free employer contributions, standardize benefit coverages within sponsored groups, risk-adjust premiums, group small employers into large health insurance purchasing cooperatives, and require production of reliable data on quality, especially as measured by outcomes" [Enthoven 1993]. Enthoven and Ellwood (hereafter referred to as Double E) understood that effective competition in the health care market could develop only if consumers became cost conscious in their choice of health care coverage. Their proposal is directed at getting a level playing field between HMOs and fee-for-service health care by intervening on the demand side to correct existing market deficiencies. They would restructure the market so that all consumers, whether in employer-sponsored or government-entitlement programs, will be motivated to consider the cost effectiveness of the alternative delivery mechanisms in choosing how to spend their health care benefit.

The Clinton adaptation of the managed competition concept shares the preference for encouraging private sector consumer enrollment in HMOs, but it does not go so far as to encourage Medicare beneficiaries to behave similarly. No HMO incentives are introduced into the Medicare program even though projected cost savings in Medicare and Medicaid are the primary source of financing the additional government entitlements, e.g., the government's 80 percent share of pre-65 retirees' premiums and the federal premium subsidies to small businesses, created by the proposal. In fact, the Clinton administration recently announced that it would not "prod elderly Medicare patients to join health maintenance organizations, in part, because they have discovered that the Government loses money on people enrolled in such private health plans" [Pear 1993c].

In the initial Clinton proposal released in September, the primary inducements for employees to consider HMOs more favorably was simply to limit the fee-for-service alternative to a single plan and to impose higher regulated premiums on that option. One of the most significant changes that was made in the legislative draft of the Clinton proposal was to permit multiple fee-for-service plans to be marketed in the area served by a regional alliance in response to objections raised by those who wished to maintain the freedom of choice of physician. Whereas Double E recognized that an artificially created advantage for HMOs would simply reduce their incentive to operate in a cost-effective manner, the Clinton proposal tried to manage the outcome of employee-consumer choice by rigging the process in the HMO's favor.

Governmental management of market outcomes is usually called regulation, not market competition. This distinction is especially clear in the change of the Health Insurance Purchasing Cooperative (HIPC) in the Jackson Hole proposal to the regional alliance in Clinton's. The original function of the HIPC had been to reduce the administrative costs and spread the insurance risks of smaller employment groups to make competition in the health insurance market fairer and more effective. However, the Clinton proposal made more than a nominal change in creating the regional alliance as its replacement for the HIPC. Despite the Clinton administration's substitution of the regional alliance for the HIPC, it has continued to employ the California Public Employees' Retirement System (CalPERS) as the singular example of how regional alliances can be successful in negotiating lower prices for health care services. In fact, CalPERS, which was the prototype organization for Enthoven's idea of HIPCs, would go out of business if the Clinton reform plan were adopted.

The regional alliance has taken on an entirely different role by becoming the regulator-purchasing agent for virtually all employment groups. Companies with more than 5,000 employees, which employ less than 10 percent of all employed Americans, have a one-time option at the inception of the program to operate their own plans without utilizing the regional alliance, but companies that choose to operate independently of the alliance forgo the protection of a federal cap on premium costs of 7.9 percent of payroll [Winslow 1993]. It has absolute authority for rate making of all fee-for-service providers, controls direct marketing to consumers by health plans, publishes information about health plans to permit consumers to make valid comparisons of the plans, and contracts with all health plans serving the area. In addition, it must impose the federal formula for fixing a ceiling on the annual rate of premium increases. The regional alliance owes a greater kinship to the Regional Offices of Health Security in Kennedy's 1970 proposal, which also had such fiscal regulatory authority, than to the Jackson Hole Group's purchasing cooperatives.

The use of an arbitrary federal ceiling on health care spending is another commonality of the Clinton and 1970 Kennedy proposals, which is the simplest conceptual method of containing health care costs, but has many unintended consequences. The Clinton plan, through its premium increase ceiling and a separate limit on the rate of Medicare expenditure increases, imposes such a limit, but it does so in the most complicated of all NHI proposals to avoid raising federal taxes. Instead the Kennedy plan proposed raising both income and payroll taxes to finance the program and fixed the spending limit by the rate of increase in financing.

The only apparent advantage of this convoluted method of financing and cost containment is to avoid a substantial federal tax increase and to dress a regulatory intervention as a competitive, market approach. The latter approach also conceals the plan's effect of transferring a sizeable portion of the government's current obligation for financing the care of the poor and the aged to the private sector without raising taxes. The Lewin-VHI study of the Clinton plan's costs confirmed that "Employers will pay a 14 percent increase in premiums to help even the costs of covering high-cost, non-working populations included in the community-rated pool" [John Sheils of Lewin as quoted in Gearon 1994]. The government's projected budget reductions for existing programs is based on the cap-induced savings and "by forcing employers to pay some costs now paid by Medicare and Medicaid" [Pear 1993b].

The community rating requirement for premiums regulated by the regional alliances has precisely that effect. However, by virtue of the Clinton reform plan for a guaranteed national benefit package for the private sector while maintaining the independence of the Medicare program, the federal government could also become the world's first oligopsonist to have the right to determine the prices that other purchasers must pay by simply removing the cap of 7.9 percent of payroll on private premium costs. Such an amendment to the program is extremely likely if Congress is faced with voter complaints about the quality and availability of health care, or should the formula ceiling of health insurance premiums ever prove insufficient to adequately finance health care services. The only other, and much less attractive, alternative available to Congress would be to raise taxes to pay for a larger subsidy for businesses' health insurance benefits.

Two process conclusions can be drawn from these comparisons:

1. From the comparison of all three plans, regulation described as managed competition is much more palatable to both the regulated and the business sector;

2. From the comparison between the 1970 Kennedy NHI proposal and Clinton's 1993 reform proposal, New Democrats appear to be better accountants than Old Democrats, at least in finding ways to increase government revenues without increasing taxes.

Confronting the Political Constraints

The Clinton administration is being devious in describing its health care reform proposal because of its conviction that the electorate is strongly opposed to any income and/or payroll tax increases as the means of financing NHI, and that the Congress shares that view. The updated version of Kennedy's 1970 proposal, now referred to as the single-payer approach and cosponsored by Representative Jim McDermott of Washington and Senator Paul D. Wellstone of Minnesota, has received support only from doctrinaire, Old Democrats, who are still advocating a social-insurance solution to NHI. This bill is given little chance of being approved by the Congress.

The Clinton plan's use of an employer mandate as the principal financing mechanism is certainly neither unprecedented nor objectionable as a means of winning congressional approval of health care reform. For instance, Senator Kennedy switched from an all-federal-tax approach 20 years ago when he cosponsored an NHI plan with Representative Wilbur Mills that was financed primarily through an employer-mandate of coverage.

What is unique about the Clinton proposal is the lengths to which the mandated approach has been taken to transfer a part of the government's financial obligation for the health care of the poor and the aged to the private sector. No previous sponsor of the mandated approach has been quite so bold, but no other sponsor has ever faced so much pressure to reduce the federal deficit. Nevertheless, burdening employers with an additional obligation for the poor and the aged beyond the tax support that is currently being provided through the Medicare payroll tax and federal general tax revenues does demonstrate that the mandating approach, i.e., a government requirement for private parties to expend funds for a particular purpose, is, indeed, a tax that does not have to be accounted for by government. Much to President Clinton's chagrin, the Congressional Budget Office has interpreted the employer mandate as a tax and thus recommended that it be included in the federal budget [Pear 1994.]

Although the interpretation is theoretically correct, as is CBO's conclusion that the plan is based on the use of sovereign power of government, no other mandate of government has ever been accounted for in the federal budget.

In the final analysis, the employees will have to bear those increased taxes, not employers [Feldman 1993]. The employees will receive lower cash wages in future negotiations as a result of the additional obligation levied on employers. As is always the case with tax questions, the issue of additional taxes is one of equity between taxpayers. Is it fair to tax employees (current workers) for both their own health insurance costs and for an additional contribution to the financing of Medicare and Medicaid? The equity issue is even more complex because the Clinton plan compels all employees, the healthy and the unhealthy, to buy the same amount of health insurance coverage and pay the same community rate for that coverage. A question of the fairness of this arrangement to the healthier worker can also be raised.

Avoiding the appearance of a direct tax increase to finance universal benefits is the first political constraint or hurdle that most congressmen have accepted as a condition for passing health care reform. The second condition is the ratchet-like constraint on government entitlement programs by which benefits can only increase, never decrease. This constraint is especially pronounced for the Medicare entitlement, which is vigorously defended by the powerful senior citizens lobby. It was President Clinton's acceptance of this constraint that led to the ingenuous design of an employer-mandate that made the employed pay for the increased cost of Medicare's additional health care benefits that are in the expanded universal package of the benefits and still propose to finance NHI with lower projected costs for Medicare and Medicaid.

Because the cost of health care for those 65 and over already constitutes more than 40 percent[23] and will be an ever larger portion of the nation's total health care bill, this constraint means that health care reform proposals cannot revise Medicare benefits or increase beneficiary responsibilities, and it limits the cost containment effort to the population under 65. Although those under 65 constitute 87 percent of the population, they only consume 60 percent of the nation's health care resources. If the aged, the fastest growing age group in the population, continue their present health care consumption pattern, the pressure for containing the health care costs of younger

Americans, who are already being asked to pay a greater share of the total bill in the Clinton plan, will intensify. This solution is neither equitable nor likely to be effective.

The third political constraint on health care reform is that no, or at least as few as possible, Americans should be asked to pay more for health insurance than is currently being paid. Because this constraint is logically impossible and contradicts the other two constraints, the Clinton administration has simply tried to conceal as much as possible the cost increase to any group. As a result, statements like Health and Human Services Secretary Donna E. Shalala's faux pas before Congress of presenting a graph showing that 40 percent of American families would pay higher premiums, have had to be denied. In the case of Shalala's testimony, an immediate "correction" was issued by the director of the Office of Management and Budget, Leon E. Panetta. He reported that only 30 percent would have higher premiums along with more health insurance coverage, and that only 1 in 1,000 would have as much as an $83 per month increase in costs while 15.1 percent of families would save more than $83 a month.

Despite such claims, it is not surprising that 70 percent of the public, as reported in an October 1993 *Washington Post* national public opinion poll [Morin and Broder 1993], expected their medical care costs to increase as a result of the Clinton plan, and 68 percent also expected their taxes to increase to pay for the reform plan. Without question, the public would prefer not to have increased taxes as the price for a universal set of portable health insurance benefits that could never be taken away. Nevertheless, there is significant ambiguity in the public's concern about higher taxes. Its desire for health security and outrage about constantly rising health care costs and unfair health insurance company practices suggests that strong political leadership, especially with bipartisan support, could persuade the public that an equitable tax increase is worthwhile. In other words, there may be sufficient benefits in the public's view of health care reform that the no-tax-increase constraint could be overcome with a good reform plan that would enhance consumer choice and reduce future health care costs.

The toughest constraint to modify, regardless of the quality of leadership, is the prohibition on materially changing the Medicare program. The aged are obviously more anxious about their health and financial security than any other segment of our population. What kind of trade-offs would give the aged benefits equivalent to or greater than first-dollar, free choice of physician, health insurance? Even if alternative benefits could be provided, it is important to remember that the current age group that is 65 and over was instilled with the value of this type of health insurance in the post-World War II era. This age group does not believe that it paid for it the way social security was paid for with a lifetime of payroll taxes. They perceive Medicare as the most vulnerable government entitlement that has been provided to this group of American citizens. That is why its enactment was so politically popular and why any proposed cost containment changes in the Medicare benefit structure can only be implemented prospectively with an ironclad assurance grandfathering this age group's benefits for the rest of their lives.

The third constraint is the easiest to overcome because few really believe the Clinton claim that practically no one under age 65 will have to pay more for health care services. Unlike the over 65 age group, the under 65's lifetime experience has been a rising percentage of family income being spent on health care, partly because this age group has been paying the payroll taxes for Medicare. The plan must, however, clearly identify those whose costs will increase further and why they may expect lower rates of health care cost increases in the future. The key to overcoming this constraint is a sound health care cost containment plan.

If the current Medicare program entitlements represent the only binding constraint on the enactment of effective health care reform legislation, the challenges that remain are strong political leadership and the development of a plan that really will contain future health care cost increases.

A REFORM PLAN REDRESSING PAST MARKET TRANSGRESSIONS

A compromise health care reform plan can be constructed by accepting, first, the Clinton bottom line of universal coverage by a noncancelable health insurance plan and, second, by eliminating the flaws in the market for health care services in the United States. Health care reform must provide universal insurance coverage for health security and correct the health insurance mechanism so that the consumer can assume the key role in making health care market decisions.

The accomplishment of those two goals will require violating to various degrees the three political constraints that the Clinton planners have held as sacrosanct—some new taxes will be required to finance universal benefits; the Medicare program must be modified prospectively for those not yet aged 65; and some individuals, in accordance with their ability to pay, will be asked to pay more for health insurance and/or services. However, the provision of health security for all delivered in a cost-effective manner can only be achieved through sacrifice of real alternatives forgone; or as Victor Fuchs stated it "if there is no pain there will be no gain" [Fuchs 1993a].

The principal deficiency in the U.S. health insurance market is an overabundance of "free" first or low dollar coverage, which has reduced consumer sacrifice but at the cost of permitting health care providers to make all of the important resource allocation decisions. The need to eliminate another major existing deficiency—the lack of any health insurance coverage for a sizeable group of the population—makes this a most propitious time for crafting a solution. The enactment of an NHI program is the most direct means of providing health insurance to all our citizens, and the careful construction of that legislation is the best way to restore the consumers' appropriate role in health care decision making.

The 1970s view that NHI can be used both to control health care costs and address the issue of access to health care was valid. However, few proposals advanced in the early '70s would have directly contained health care costs because most plans were based on the same first or low dollar insurance premise that has disrupted rational marketplace decision making in health care and sought to impose government regulation, rather than market reform, to contain health care costs. Their efforts demonstrated the futility of regulation and made market reform the preferred solution in the '90s.

The primary reason for the failure of health care regulation to control health care costs is the unwillingness of government regulators to stand up to health care providers when the electorate has no stake (receives no direct benefit) in health care cost savings. To the contrary, successful regulatory cost containment threatens the availability and/ or quality of health care services that are virtually "free" to health care consumers—the voters. What rational elected or appointed government official will go to the mat fighting for a cost containment goal that is likely to offend the voters?

Successful health care reform, whether employing a market or regulatory approach, must give the voters/consumers a stake (positive benefits) in health care cost containment. The advantage of a market approach to reform is its superiority for directly involving the people in controlling health care costs because they can see the benefits of lower costs directly in the most tangible way—the amount of money they have left for other goods and services.

The alternative reform proposal, therefore, employs an approach that seeks to correct the existing insurance defects in the health care market, which are described historically in the next section. The eradication of those defects—too much first-dollar coverage and discrimination against high-risk persons—requires an upside down rebuilding of the health insurance market through the provision of a limited social insurance benefit by the federal government. The tax financing of that benefit is described and followed by a general statement of consumer options in the transformed health insurance market. Penultimately, the administration of the NHI program, which is generally consistent with the Clinton framework of a National Health Board supervising state program administration, is described. Finally, the implications of the insurance market changes and the greater consumer role in the purchase of health care are discussed. Exactly how health care providers will respond to the revitalized consumer direction cannot be controlled as precisely as President Clinton and the advocates of managed competition believe, but given proper incentives for cost effective, efficacious health care, an innovative competitive process will meet consumer needs and contain health care costs.

The Actuaries' 1930s Definition of the Problem

One means of constructing an effective market reform proposal is to review the period when health insurance in the United States went astray and ask how the health insurance mechanism could have been designed to overcome the subsequent problems of first-dollar coverage and the guaranteed freedom of choice of physician. Ironically, these questions were asked by the commercial insurance actuaries during the development of the health insurance product in the 1930s. Actuaries from commercial insurance carriers then questioned whether health care was insurable for two reasons: (1) those in poorer health were more likely to purchase insurance than healthier individuals so health insurance sales would be to a group of the population that was less healthy than the uninsured population, and (2) once insurance coverage was obtained, regardless of the individual's health, the coverage would encourage greater utilization of health care services than the individual would have consumed without coverage.

As the history of the health care market has demonstrated these early insurance actuaries' concerns were valid. The actuaries were correct that illness was not randomly distributed across the population. In fact, most Americans are quite healthy, have few illnesses over their lifetimes, and have relatively low total health care costs over their entire lives. A sizeable minority has a significant amount of illness and incur substantial health care costs, and less than 10 percent have very serious health problems and will experience extraordinary health care costs during their lives. Therefore, from the insurers standpoint, it was important that insurance sales plans minimize the opportunity for individual choice because individual choice would have resulted in a disproportionate number of the higher risk individuals buying insurance. The fortuitous development of group plans at place of employment with employer premium subsidization was ideal for the insurers because nearly all of the healthier individuals were included in the group. Subsequently private insurers adopted techniques, like the preexisting condition provision, for excluding the higher risk individuals from the group to lower their loss ratios.

From the consumer's standpoint the highly favorable distribution of the incidence of illness has been perverted through the prevalence of employer-sponsored first dollar, free choice, health insurance. The healthy half of the population has bought far too much health insurance, assuming that the alternative to all that insurance would have been higher rates of cash wage increases. Even with such good odds and the knowledge that a person's state of health has a high degree of stability over a lifetime, some health insurance would have been a sound investment for peace of mind and financial security. Everyone is aware of friends or relatives who have suffered from poor health and incurred high costs of illness or accident. However, the kind of coverage that would have been appropriate for most healthy individuals would have been a high deductible or last-dollar coverage, which is much less costly than first-dollar insurance and could have resulted in higher take-home pay.

The actuaries were correct that in a market where individuals exercised rational choice only the less healthy individuals or families and the highly risk averse would have purchased the first-dollar type of health insurance. However, in the United States through a series of wartime happenstances first-dollar with free choice of physician became practically the only form of health insurance in the market until the 1980s surge of managed care organizations. In other words, the principal flaw in the health insurance market is that health insurance started at the wrong end of the coverage continuum, and that flaw became ingrained in the health care market by the imprinting of consumers after World War II and by the Congress in 1965 with the passage of Medicare-Medicaid legislation. Only after that action did health care costs in the United States go out of control in comparison with such costs in other developed nations.

The overpurchase of health insurance affirmed the actuaries' second concern—having insurance will increase the insured's utilization of health care services. Further, the design of the dominant form of insurance could not have been worse. First-dollar coverage by itself is inflationary, but when coupled with freedom of choice of physician, the results can be explosively inflationary as demonstrated by Medicare. Without any additional cost controls, Medicare and Medicaid covered those most in need of health services, the poor and the aged, and changed the demand for health care well beyond the function of meeting only the individual consumer's medical needs.

The out-of-pocket consumer costs for health care services became totally unrelated to the total cost of these services. Consumers, with little direct consequence, were satisfied to let the physicians decide what and how these services should be provided. Thus, physicians can practice the kind of scientific medicine that they had been taught to admire in medical school with little regard for its cost. As a result, too many cesarean rather than vaginal births have occurred, too many prostatectomies have been performed instead of watchingful waiting, and too many coronary artery bypass grafts have been made instead of trying less invasive procedures. Where less invasive diagnostic technologies, such as ultrasound or constantly improving imaging services, have become available, they have been overprescribed. There are twice as many specialists in the United States as suggested by the pattern of practice in other developed countries. The cost of following the physician's preference, without any economically concerned consumer challenge, for this high-tech, specialized style of care is not insignificant. Both the 1982 Rand Study and the international comparisons in chapter 5 suggest that the cost of excess health care utilization is approximately 30 percent of current health care spending in the United States, about $300 billion in 1994.

Turning Health Insurance Upside Down

Health insurance should be available to all Americans to finance medically needed health care services without encouraging the purchase of unnecessary services. What's needed is an insurance mechanism that is activated when individuals or families have health care needs that are beyond their ability to finance the same way they purchase other important consumer goods and services. Last-dollar coverage, not first-dollar, is needed to correct the flaw in the health insurance market. Further, such coverage is the most appropriate for social insurance; i.e., the distribution of expected losses is concentrated on only a few persons or families, and the federal government is the appropriate body to spread these risks as broadly as possible.

If the federal government had insured the unaffordable-last-dollar of health care costs, as defined in this way, as part of the 1935 Social Security Act, the health insurance market in the United States would have developed appropriately with effective competition in the health care market. The sale of first-dollar coverage would have been limited to a small segment of less healthy and especially risk sensitive persons. The incentive for health insurance carriers and integrated health care providers to avoid enrolling high-risk persons would have been eliminated because the federal government would insure those persons with unaffordable health care costs. The health care market would have developed like other markets in which consumers are sensitive to the price of services. The Rand Study demonstrated that families above the poverty level would *not* have failed to purchase needed health care services with such insurance protection [Brooks et al 1983].

The appropriate time for the government to assist an individual or a family is when the health care costs are beyond their ability to finance needed services. Financing implies paying for those services out of cash reserves or borrowing the cash to pay the health care provider and, after receiving the service, paying back the loan, which describes how consumers currently pay for other goods and services. The ability of a family to finance health services or any service, for that matter, is primarily determined by the level of the family's income.

Therefore, to ensure that all Americans will be able to purchase needed health services, the federal government would have to define unaffordable health losses in terms of the family's income. For example, the first dollar of health care costs for a family whose income is below the poverty level is an unaffordable loss, but for a millionaire the unaffordable loss might not occur until several hundred thousand dollars of health care costs have been incurred.

If last dollar health insurance coverage was provided by the federal government, high risk persons would largely become the financial responsibility of the federal insurance program. Consequently, insurance carriers would no longer have any incentive to inappropriately limit preexisting conditions, and this practice as well as other more subtle exclusions would be abandoned in a competitive market for insurance premiums revenues. Nor would the carriers have to charge higher premiums to smaller groups and individuals because there would no longer be a greater likelihood of higher catastrophic risks. The level of liability that would be insured in the private health insurance market would be capped and the federal government would become the insurer of last resort.

A federal health insurance program covering unaffordable costs would be a true social insurance program. It would define the benefits in terms of the citizen's ability to pay for health care costs instead of a fixed dollar amount, as the deductibles in most health insurance benefits packages are currently structured. Rice and Thorpe [1993] make a very persuasive case for income-related cost sharing; they note that "Because cost-sharing requirements are usually unrelated to ability to pay, they can be very regressive" and that because a higher proportion of the lower-income population are in poorer health, "this problem is exacerbated." The most equitable (and easiest to administer) definition would be to define the benefit in terms of percentage of (taxable) family income spent on specified health care goods and services.

The criteria for establishing the percentage should be threefold: (1) what a family could reasonably be expected to plan for and finance out of its own resources (including contributions from employers for health insurance); (2) what the federal government can afford to finance in a fiscally responsible manner that is acceptable to the various classes of taxpayers; and (3) what level of spending by families will constitute a sufficient deterrent to unnecessary health care without inhibiting the provision of necessary health care services.

One of the NHI proposals in the 1970s was Martin Feldstein's [Eilers and Moyerman 1971], which recommended that the federal government provide last-dollar coverage to all citizens and also provide a government-guaranteed program of post-care loans to assist in financing the deductible and copayment provisions of the coverage. Feldstein suggested that the deductible be established at 5 percent of family income followed by a 50 percent copayment on the next 10 percent of family income; i.e., the total health care expenditures could not be higher than 10 percent of family income, but they would receive a federal benefit of 50 percent of health expenditures after spending 5 percent of their income. He recommended an exception for members of families below the federally-defined poverty level of income, who should be made eligible for the first dollar, i.e., a zero deductible, of health care spending.

Obviously, the percentages of deductible and copayments could be changed for segments of the population, e.g., lower-income persons above the poverty line might have a lower deductible and higher-income persons might have an even higher copayment percentage, or the basic percentage could be raised or lowered depending on subjective agreement on the three criteria identified earlier. For the sake of illustration in the remainder of this discussion, it will be assumed that the Feldstein proposal does satisfy these criteria; along with a requirement that, to reduce the insurance incentive for excess utilization, private insurers limit their low-dollar coverage to a minimum of, say, a deductible of 1 percent of family income and some reasonable level of copayment, say 20 percent of the remaining health care expenditures up to 9 percent of its family income.

There is a possible problem of insurance-induced utilization for the poverty-level families and the catastrophically-ill, who, after reaching the deductible limit, also have "free" health care. However, the use of deductibles and coinsurance is inappropriate for both groups. One method for the poor would be to require HMO participation to qualify for the "free" health care services. An appropriate government agency could seek competitive bids from area HMOs to care for specific numbers of poor families living in the area. As much as possible, individual poor families should have a choice of the local HMOs. To prevent developing a separate health care system for the poor, the number of poor families could be limited in terms of the ratio of poor to nonpoor registrants in the participating HMOs.

The problem of excess utilization of health care services by the catastrophically ill is especially difficult, however, and a variety of approaches will be required to find the best solutions. Each state will have to develop a plan for monitoring and controlling the health care costs of the catastrophically ill. Special program incentives may be developed for health care providers to find innovative programs for caring these patients. Alternatively, regulation and/or rationing of particular treatment regimens may be required. Although there are no guaranteed solutions, experimentation and a focus on the appropriateness of treatment for these patients may lead to better and more economical care. Under the current insurance schemes, these patients are avoided, not singled out for special attention.

Financing Federal Last-Dollar Benefits

Some general determination must be made about the method of financing the new federal last-dollar benefits. "Government policy toward health care can never be separated from financing or tax issues, or from alternative uses and expenditures to which tax dollars might be devoted. In many discussions, health policy is treated as isolated from tax policy. Inevitably and irreducibly, however, they are two sides of the same accounting ledger" [C. Eugene Steuerie by Pear 1993a]. Although Steuerie's observation complicates the problem, finding acceptable tax revenue sources to finance a new federal benefit is a necessary prerequisite for the approval of health care reform, especially in the 1990s.

As the discussion in chapters 3 and 5 demonstrated, one of the major causes of the dysfunctional growth of first or low-dollar health insurance coverage in the post-World War II period was the policy decision to exempt employer-provided health insurance from federal income taxation. President Reagan's proposals for tax reform in 1986 included either the elimination of or caps on the tax exemption of health insurance benefits, but Senator Robert Packwood of Oregon, who was chairman of the Senate Finance Committee and the congressional champion of the health insurance exemption, blocked its inclusion in the final draft of the bill [Birnbaum and Murray, 1987]. In 1992 that exemption cost the federal government $63 billion in tax revenues, according to federal estimates [Pear 1993a]. The elimination of the exemption could provide the principal source of revenue for universal coverage of unaffordable health care costs.

The incremental cost to the federal government of such a universal program may not be as great as many would expect because the vast majority of the catastrophically ill are lower-income and aged persons who are currently covered through the Medicare and Medicaid programs. The federal government's responsibility for the poor, the disabled, and the aged suggests that most catastrophically-ill persons are already included in government insurance programs. For example, Berk and Monheit [1992] estimate that in 1987 nearly 65 percent of the persons in the top 1 percent of health care expenditures were over 65 (48.2 percent) or black (16.3 percent). Because race has proven to be a good proxy for low income status, the 40 percent higher representation of blacks in the top 1 percent spending category than in the general population is indicative that more lower income persons are in this category also.

As stated earlier, these new benefits are not a politically acceptable replacement for the current beneficiaries of the Medicare program, but the new benefits program could be phased in by stopping new Medicare enrollments for persons who become 65 after the new benefits become available. To assure the current Medicare beneficiaries that the reform proposal will help them, the benefits eligible for the unaffordable limit on expenditures should be added to the Medicare program benefits. The expenditure limit should also be made available to Medicare beneficiaries for out-of-pocket health care expenditures exceeding the 10 percent of the family income of the 65 and older to provide some additional assistance to the lower-income aged. In designing these additional benefits for Medicare, some cost containment incentives might be introduced; for example, requiring the recipient to join an HMO enrollment or give up Medigap insurance in order to qualify for the additional last-dollar coverage. Both for reasons of equity and for raising additional tax revenues, the actuarial value of Medicare benefits ought also be subject to the federal income tax, but that step would require stronger political leadership than can be expected in the current environment.

If the increased tax revenues on personal income are not sufficient to balance the increased cost of the new social insurance for the federal government, there is merit in encouraging a more healthy lifestyle for Americans through Clinton's proposal to raise the so-called "sin" taxes on tobacco. President Clinton excluded alcohol from his sin tax because of congressional opposition. However, excess alcohol consumption is one of the most serious life-style behaviors that causes serious health problems and increased costs. In addition, during the implementation of the program and before all of the potential savings in health care costs that will result from the restructured and more effective marketplace, say the first five years, the federal government could require state governments to pay a declining percentage of their reduced obligations for Medicaid program costs that will be replaced by the new program. That is, state governments will be relieved of sharing in the cost of Medicaid. It is proposed that they be asked to contribute to the federal government their Medicaid appropriations in the year before the commencement of the new program in the first year, 80 percent in the programs second year, 60, 40 and 20 percent in the three succeeding years.

Taxing individuals for employer-provided health insurance on the health care market would go a long way toward restoring the consumer's cost consciousness in health care decision making. Strengthening the health care marketplace, and a significant source of stimulus to economic expansion, could be achieved by giving each employee with a health insurance benefit the option of taking the employer's contribution partially or in whole as cash wages in the year that these benefits become taxable. In 1987 more than 60 percent of two-worker families were both offered employer-sponsored coverage and 63 percent of those families accept coverage from two different employers [Shur and Taylor 1991]. It is proposed that during the implementation year two-worker families choose which member is to receive the health benefit, and the other receives a salary increase equal to the value of the earned health benefit. At the time of conversion, employees should receive compensation for all previously earned benefits. Thereafter changes in all health insurance fringes will be negotiated as a part of the total wage package. Employers should accept this additional cost as a buy-out of a constantly rising health insurance obligation. The new federal benefit will also substantially reduce the employers' obligation for the health insurance of retired employees, but not by as much as the Clinton proposal.

In addition to giving employees the option to take the employer's contribution to health insurance premiums in either continued premium payments or increased take-home pay, all employers would be mandated, much as in Representative Jim Cooper' reform proposal, to serve as administrative agents for employee purchases of health insurance benefits by making available multiple insurance options, including both fee-for-service and HMO coverage. After the first year of the program, the employers would not be responsible for paying any increased premium costs unless changes are a part of labor negotiations or voluntary agreement.

The Consumer's Option—Benefits versus Take-Home Pay

The availability of last-dollar health insurance for all Americans would change the consumer's choice of specific private health insurance alternatives that would be purchased either through the citizen's employer or directly by the family. The proposal would make available to all citizens a portable set of last-dollar benefits, regardless of where or even if they were employed, that should eliminate the existing fear of personal bankruptcy resulting from illness or accident. In addition, it will reduce the cost of a lower-dollar private health insurance coverage or HMO enrollment that consumers might wish to purchase.

It is assumed that most citizens, whose family incomes exceed the federal definition of poverty, ($6,932 for one person and $13,924 for a family of four in 1991) will probably want to at least consider covering the 5 percent of family-income deductible and the 50 percent copayment on the next 9 percent of family income by purchasing additional health insurance or enrolling in an HMO. Either arrangement could cover most (up to 1 percent of the deductible and the 20 percent copayment on the remainder) of the federal deductible and copayment requirements. That is, the higher-risk protection is not necessarily intended to be a substitute for comprehensive health insurance benefits, but it could serve as the foundation upon which consumers can build a broader health security program within the boundaries defining the individual's and the government's responsibilities.

The purpose of this section is to demonstrate that most Americans will benefit substantially from federal protection against unaffordable health care costs financed by income taxes imposed on individuals' employer-provided health insurance and to focus on the income groups that will be most affected by the tax increase and the choice of whether to self-insure or continue to purchase health insurance below the catastrophic level. This accounting of how the American people would fare from the catastrophic health proposal is based on 1991 data as compiled by Levit et al [1992]. Because health insurance coverage has declined since that time, the effect on Americans is actually better, i.e., more people would benefit, than these numbers indicate.

The Categorical Winners

Many Americans would benefit from this reform proposal because they would receive catastrophic health insurance protection without any direct or immediate cost. The most obvious beneficiaries are the 34.7 million Americans who currently have no health insurance. They would receive the protection of a health spending limit of 5 percent of their income plus 50 percent of 10 percent of their income without any increase in federal income taxes. In addition, many of the employed who are currently without insurance, nearly 27 million of the uninsured, would have the opportunity to purchase insurance to cover 72 percent of this deductible at a much lower cost than is presently available. More than half the American labor force works for firms with fewer than 100 employees, and a much larger percentage of these employees are uninsured. Therefore, a reduction in small groups' premiums could be a significant inducement for the purchase of private insurance or HMO enrollment. Individuals and small groups are currently assessed much higher premiums than members of larger groups because of the risk of enrolling individuals who are in poorer health and the inability to spread these higher costs in the smaller plans. However, making the federal government the insurer of last resort for catastrophic illness should substantially lower permium costs to small groups and individuals who are not eligible for any group enrollment.

The second large group of beneficiaries are individuals who currently purchase health insurance themselves, the self-employed, the early retirees who are not yet eligible for Medicare, and the employed who are purchasing their own insurance without assistance from their employer. About 15 million persons in this group are under 65 years of age, according Levit et al. [1992]. All members of this group, depending on their particular income level, will receive a substantial drop in their health insurance premiums if they wish to continue coverage of the federal deductible or they can obtain even larger savings if they wish to self-insure that deductible. Most of those who are purchasing their own health insurance probably have a major medical policy and, unless they are members of an insurance group, are likely to be paying a minimum of $3,600 to $4,000 a year, but premiums of $10,000 to $12,000 are not unheard of for high-risk families (i.e., families who have experienced serious health problems). These individuals would be the biggest winners because they would obtain these additional benefits and a substantial reduction, depending on their level of family income, for private health insurance if they choose to continue their private insurance or HMO coverage for the federal deductible and copayment provisions. In general, the higher the premiums that they are currently paying and the lower their family income, the greater the savings will be, but even those families earning at or near median incomes and paying the lower premiums should receive substantial premium reductions. Further, except for the smokers in this group, there will be no additional taxes for the catastrophic insurance benefits. One of the secondary benefits of this change in the health insurance market will be the removal of an impediment to the early retirement of employees who wish to retire but are currently discouraged by the high cost of health insurance.

The third group of categorical winners are those families living at or below the poverty level, some 30 million under age 65 and 3.7 million who are 65 or older. With the zero deductible for persons living below the poverty level, this program would be a significant improvement over the existing Medicaid program. In addition, only 24.3 million were eligible for Medicaid in 1991. Consequently, 9.4 million persons would become eligible for first-dollar health insurance coverage, an even greater improvement in health insurance benefits than the general improvement in Medicaid benefits.

The last group that would receive federal protection at no additional cost are the Medicare beneficiaries at the time the new program goes into operation. They would continue their existing benefits and receive a catastrophic limit on their out-of-pocket health expenditures including prescription drugs and some long-term care benefits. The existing Medicare benefits should not be changed, but the new benefits for prescription drugs and assistance with long-term care should qualify for the catastrophic coverage, which limits the benefit to those chronically ill aged requiring these services. There are slightly more than 26 million aged whose incomes are above the poverty level and are eligible for Medicare, and another 1.2 million disabled would receive these additional benefits.

In total in 1991, about 110 million Americans, some 44.4 percent of the population, would have received substantial assistance from the federal last-dollar health insurance program without any additional taxes, except for the smokers in this group. Further, most of these Americans are in the lower-income population who have a higher probability of health care need and benefit most from additional health care.

Employees with Health Insurance Benefits

The 138 million Americans who are covered by employer-sponsored health insurance coverage would finance the catastrophic coverage for all Americans. Although it may be argued that this is just retribution for the half century of tax subsidies that have been granted to these employees, retribution is rarely a politically acceptable rationale for a public policy change. The retroactive imposition of the 1993 tax increase for upper-income Americans is a notable exception to this rule. Instead of retribution the rationale is based on equity between taxpayers and the implications for the effectiveness of the nation's health care system: why should only some employees be granted tax-free health insurance benefits and be encouraged to bid up health care prices for those employees who have to pay for health care services out of after-tax income?

Even with a valid policy rationale for taxing health insurance benefits, there is a political need to demonstrate that most of those Americans who will be subject to higher taxes will receive comparable or greater benefits from the new federal last-dollar program that will result from the increased taxes. Those taxpayers who will receive net benefits from the program are in the lower tax brackets and the healthier upper-income Americans who have been buying too much health insurance in the past.

First of all, it is easy to show that most middle-income employees will receive net positive benefits (higher take-home pay and sufficient health insurance coverage at substantially lower cost) by looking at the net health service costs by income level. Table 7.1 shows the personal liability for the mean income of each income category, which is 10 percent of the mean family income; the net personal liability, i.e. the minimum liability for out-of-pocket expenses that would have to be borne—a deductible of 1 percent of family income plus a 20 percent copayment on expenditures up to 9 percent of family income— by each family; and the remaining personal liability for which insurance could be purchased, 7.2 percent of family income. For example, consider a family or individual earning $30,000. With that level of income, the federal catastrophic insurance would cover all health expenditures over $3,000, 10 percent of family income which repre-

TABLE 7.1   Residual Private Liabilities with Federal Last-Dollar Insurance

Income Groups	Personal Liability	Net Personal Liability	Insurable Liability
0—$15K	$ 1,100*	$ 308	$ 792
$15–25K	2,000	560	1,440
$25–35K	3,000	840	2,160
$35–50K	4,250	1,190	3,060
$50–75K	6,250	1,750	4,500
$75–100K	8,250	2,310	5,940
$100–150K	12,500	3,500	9,000
$150–200K	17,500	4,900	12,600

*Most families in this income category would qualify for full federal coverage with no deductible, but individuals earning more than $7,000 would be subject to the respective liabilities shown in this line.

sents the maximum personal liability of the family, column 1. The family could purchase private health insurance that would cover its residual liability after paying a deductible of $300, 1 percent of family income, and 20 percent copayments on the next $2,700 (9 percent of family income) or a total of $540 in copayments for a maximum out-of-pocket expense of $840, column 2. Thus, the private insurer of this family's health expenditures would have a maximum potential liability of $2,160, column 3. The premium for such a policy should be substantially less than the $2,891[24] average employers paid in the wholesale/retail industry in 1991. An employee could pay the $810 (28 percent of $2,891) in increased taxes and still purchase low-dollar comprehensive health insurance to, at least, break even.

Because higher paying industries also tend to pay larger health insurance premiums, most employees earning up to $50,000 are likely to be able to purchase the maximum private coverage at close to break even. Two-worker families with both receiving employer-provided health insurance benefits earning up to mid-$80,000 could not only break even, but substantially increase net take-home pay. More than 40 percent of all families whose family income is less than $75,000, had two workers and, because 84 percent of all employees had some employer-provided health insurance benefits, about one-third of these families should qualify for increased take-home pay when given the option to switch from health insurance to increased salaries. A conservative estimate is that virtually all families earning $15,000 to $35,000 and one-third of the families (the two-worker family) between $35,000 and $75,000 could at least break even while maintaining low-dollar health insurance coverage, and many could have an increase in take-home pay. That family estimate translates into approximately 94 of the 139 million covered by employer-sponsored health insurance.

Thus, more than 200 million of the nation's total 1991 population of 248 million, more than 80 percent, would have some positive benefit, and about two-thirds of those receiving some tax increases could continue most of their low-dollar coverage and either break even or increase their take-home pay. However, the primary purpose of reforming the health insurance market is not to continue the status quo. Enabling the middle and upper middle class employee to maintain low-dollar coverage without increasing the premium cost is, nevertheless, a political requirement for making the proposal acceptable.

Changing Consumer Behavior

The major objective of this health insurance reform proposal is to provide alternative mechanisms or incentives to the healthier non-poor working family to consider purchasing less health insurance so that these families will be sufficiently cost conscious for the health care market to operate effectively. An effective market expands consumer choices and should lead to a more satisfied public in America.

Few economists have understood the American infatuation with first-dollar coverage, its higher administrative cost, and its incentives to increase medical care utilization and cost. Fuchs has suggested that it is almost as if these consumers wished to exclude any cost consideration from their health care consumption decisions, at least in the case of major medical interventions. He theorized that this behavior could be a form of precommitment, which is "a rational strategy for dealing with problems of self-control . . . when there is tension between alternative behaviors which have very different implications for our welfare in the short and long run" [Fuchs 1979]. In other words, people are concerned that they might economize when they should be spending for care of their loved ones or themselves. Therefore, they buy excessive amounts of insurance to avoid making incorrect patient care decisions on the basis of false economy.

Last-dollar coverage is designed to provide ample safeguards to ensure that whenever major medical interventions are needed the federal government, as insurer of last resort, will provide the necessary resources. The loan-guarantee program also represents an intermediate safeguard to ensure that having cash balances available is not a prerequisite for purchasing less major forms of medical or health care services. By prospectively fixing the individual family's maximum out-of-pocket health care expenditure in any given year and providing loan guarantees, the proposal seeks to give consumers greater flexibility in planning for the purchase and financing of unexpected health care needs. It is, however, based on the fundamental premise that those consumers who can should purchase health care as wisely as they purchase other goods and services to get the most for their money.

Improving the consumer's ability to make wise health care decisions is much more likely to occur in a freely competitive market than in a managed competition or limited choice market in which "250 million morons called U.S. citizens . . . [will be] moved out, . . . their influence [reduced] and . . . smart professionals buy it on our behalf" [Kenneth S. Abramowitz as quoted by Kosterlitz 1992c]. Americans are learning that when someone else is paying the bill decisions are often made in terms of the payer's interests, not in the consumer's best interests. William Neikirk [1993] reports that "Consumers Union is so concerned about undertreatment [in managed care organizations] that it wants patients to be able to appeal denials or delays in care outside their health plans." If a freely competitive market in health care can be developed, consumers may wish to purchase their own independent professional advice for difficult medical problems.

Fortunately, most Americans will only rarely have to make difficult medical decisions, but in a restructured insurance market every citizen without a federal entitlement for low-dollar coverage will be asked to choose, either directly or by inaction, a method of obtaining health care and a means of financing the precatastrophic deductible. In assessing the likelihood and amount of health financing that may be needed, each consumer's own health record and the family's demographics are the best predictors of future needs and the appropriateness of membership in an organized delivery system like an HMO or the purchase of low-dollar coverage from a private insurance carrier. Purchasing low-dollar coverage for the deductible will be only one of several available financing options, and it is likely to be one of the more expensive alternatives.

A new option that most certainly will be offered is a savings account with the fiscal agent in which prepayments for health care services can be made and out of which the deductible can be paid when the care need arises. If no action is taken, the loan-guarantee program will be available for those who are short of cash when a health care need occurs. The essential point is that the consumer should be aware that routine health care can be paid for in a variety of ways; but regardless of the method chosen, the ultimate source of the funds is the consumer's own after-tax income.

In that sense, perhaps all Americans can be winners under a new federal program because all families with incomes above the poverty level should consider the self-insurance option with the understanding that the cost of low-dollar health insurance in the restructured insurance market will now be paid for by giving up after-tax income. With this real cost for the alternative of health insurance, the consumer will be required to consider health care service options in terms of forgoing alternative uses of personal income. There will be some pain, especially for higher-income families, but there can be gain in reduced health care costs in a reformed health care delivery system that will be much more responsive to consumer preferences.

Administration of the Program

A federal last-dollar insurance program could be administered through an organizational structure much like the one in the Clinton reform proposal, but less complex and without the regional alliances. That is, a national health board (NHB) could be established to oversee the program and monitor the performance of state governments. The states would be asked to designate a single agency to make sure that the state's American citizens and legal resident aliens receive their federal benefits. In addition, the designated state agency would be responsible for developing a comprehensive state plan for monitoring and, if approved by the NHB, regulating health care costs; proposing incentives or regulatory changes for increasing the number of health professionals, including nurse practitioners,[25] available to provide primary care; a plan for the management of care to the catastrophically ill, and a program for approving and monitoring health care financing assistance agencies (HCFAAs).

The NHB would have the authority to approve several different types of state experiments with both the financing and regulation of health care delivery as long as free and relatively unregulated competition is also given a fair trial in the majority of the states. The purpose of this experimentation is both to benchmark the effectiveness of unconstrained competition and to avoid the colossal error that has sometimes marked major federal program interventions and entitlements. Managed competition with the mandated purchase of health insurance by individuals would be an excellent experiment that perhaps Florida, Hawaii, and Washington would like to undertake. Other states, perhaps Vermont, may want to experiment with the single-payer, social insurance approach to NHI. As long as the experimenting states develop a protocol that protects their residents' federal catastrophic benefits, protects the federal government from additional costs, and obtains the appropriate state legislative authorization for the remainder of the financing, the NHB should be very permissive to learn more about ways to provide more cost-effective, efficacious health care in the United States.

The HCFAAs can also assume a variety of roles so long as they meet the underlying responsibility to their registrants to ensure that the federal government is billed for all federally qualified limits on health care expenditures and that it performs all due diligence to collect all sums owed it by its registrants.[26] It is proposed that this new agency be given great latitude to compete in the marketplace by offering a variety of services to its registrants for whom it serves as agent. In competing for registrants, the HCFAAs can offer a number of additional services such as:

1. All the managed care functions in the current market, i.e., negotiating prices with health care providers, assuming the delimited risk function for registrants' expenditures below the catastrophic limit, serving as cooperative purchasing agents for smaller employers, etc.
2. Full integration of health care delivery and financing in the staff or closed panel group practice HMOs, which, as the next section demonstrates, could be much smaller and more truly local organizations than the Clinton proposal implies unless market competition demonstrates that economies of scale would permit larger organizations to operate at lower cost.
3. Multiple financing/information functions for registrants who wish to self-insure for the deductible below the catastrophic liability of the federal government, e.g., the HCFAAs could compete solely on financial terms for the credit that is implicit in the self-insurance, or the HCFAAs could offer information about fee-for-service providers (pricing as well as professional credentials) and/or treatment options by making available

panels of professional experts to provide registrants with health care advice. (Note that some HMOs may even wish to offer independent professional review services to assure HMO registrants that they are receiving all the care that is necessary.)

The legislation should encourage the market for financing health care to develop with as much innovation as possible. The whole purpose of the reform is to put the consumer in charge of making health care consumption decisions, which has not occurred for so long that no one knows exactly what kinds of assistance will be needed. This approach is the antithesis of managed competition, which is based on the premise that the optimal organization of the health care is known and the role of reform is to lock that organizational scheme into place. Rather than calling it "unmanaged competition," which it is, perhaps "innovative competition" is a better term.

The Other Side of the Last-Dollar "Coin"

The availability of the expenditure limit will help consumers to make their health care financing decisions by limiting the extent of their liability, which also has a great psychological benefit in providing security. The more significant change in consumer behavior in the health care market will result from the manner in which the new benefits are financed—taxation of employer-provided health insurance. Such taxation will dispel the illusion of "free" health care that has been held by consumers since employer-paid health insurance was offered as an employee-recruitment inducement during World War II. Putting the value of health insurance on the employee's W–2 form will make the consumer cost conscious about health care services. *The recognition that take-home pay could be increased by lowering personal health care expenditures is the key in altering consumer health care behavior.*

Federal last-dollar health insurance may have more direct significance for health care providers/financers than for health care consumers. The availability of an expenditure limit will give health care insurers and providers the means for responding to the consumers demand for lower costs. The federal government's limiting of consumer health care liability also limits provider risk by accepting greater economic responsibility for the consumer's care. The other side of the last-dollar "coin" is the delimiting of provider risk by the federal government's providing stop loss insurance, on an individual family basis, to health care organizations willing to offer comprehensive health services to all residents of a defined service area. Health care organizations will finally have the economic and risk-bearing capabilities to integrate the delivery and financing of health care services.

As was seen earlier in the discussion of health insurance, last-dollar coverage would substantially reduce the price of individual or small group health insurance coverage. Similarly on the supply side of the market, much smaller organizations will be able to organize and market health care services on a capitation basis without concern about enrolling high-risk families. These smaller organizations, which could even consist of a medium-sized hospital and its medical staff contracting with a tertiary care organization for referral services at a preferred price, and a bank or insurance company for administrative and financing support should have many competitive advantages over larger, more bureaucratic organizations in the health care marketplace. They can provide more personalized services, adapt more quickly to local community circumstances, and avoid any substantial cost disadvantages because there is no evidence of any appreciable economies of scale in health care delivery.

Thus, both the demand and supply sides of the health care market will be substantially altered by federal last-dollar insurance as the new underpinning for health insurance. The consumer's newly created cost consciousness will interact with the provider's newly liberated ability to reorganize health care services in response to more competitive market controls. These competitive controls, through the dynamics of market interactions, will focus on the physician—the only actor in the health care marketplace that functions both as an agent for patients (consumers) and as a primary supplier and director of health care services.

J.M. Clark's "mutual compulsion" that will force all participants in the health care industry—hospitals, doctors, and insurers—"to do what no one of them would choose to do if competition did not compel them . . . . If competition did not exercise this kind of coercion, it would never reduce prices, weed out inefficient producers, and apply the spur of ruthless necessity to the others, all for the benefit of the public" [Clark 1939, 136]. In the restructured health insurance and service markets, the key question is how will this newly energized mutual compulsion affect the behavior of physicians, who control the lion's share of health care expenditures.

So far the health care industry has lacked any mutual compulsion among physicians, which resulted in the overspecialization of physician resources because they were able to choose their specialty without regard for economic consequences. The ability of many different kinds of entities to form comprehensive health care organizations and offer services on a capitated basis coupled with the consumer's need to reduce health care costs will significantly alter the demand for physicians services and, for the first time, impose economic consequences on physicians. In the fee-for-service practice of medicine, those fees will more frequently be made directly to the physician's patients and will less often be made to an abstract third party to which game playing is an acceptable part of the payment process. These changes are also part of the "pain" of health care reform to which Fuchs referred in the quote earlier in this chapter.

If the competitive market causes the expected growth of integrated health delivery organizations and/or if a more cost conscious consumer in the fee-for-service system is unwilling to pay the higher fees of specialists, then many more primary care physicians than are currently available in the marketplace will be sought. Thus, the price of primary care physician services and of nurse practitioners, however they are paid, will rise while the price for services of various medical specialties will fall. The fall may be more precipitious because of the glut of specialists and the enhanced bargaining power of the integrated health care delivery organizations and independent consumers.

The historical analogy to the excess supply of physician specialists is the price competition among hospitals in the '80s, which was more effective in markets with more competitive alternative facilities [Robinson and Luft 1988]. In addition, the physician-organized entrepreneurial services, such as surgicenters and other diagnostic and treatment centers, may in the post-reform era need to find ways to integrate with more comprehensive health care delivery organizations or go out of business, as many hospitals had to do.

When consumers are required to spend their own after-tax dollars for health care, their preferences may be satisfied in entirely different ways. For example, chronically ill patients may seek care through more specialized rather than more comprehensive organizations or younger families may select primary care organizations, and the restructuring of the health care market will follow an entirely different direction than recent trends would suggest. Regardless, the end product of health care reform will be a major reorganization and restructuring of health care services. The provision of last-dollar health insurance to all Americans, financed through a tax on employer-provided health insurance, will trigger such reform. In many ways, the resulting revolution in health care will be more unpredictable than other reform proposals because it seeks to foster free competition in the health care services market; competition that will at least initially play out in local markets without large purchasing groups acting as brokers between employers and health care delivery organzations.

One of the principal effects of the unmanaged or the innovative competition approach is to liberate employers from their role in the purchase of health insurance except to perform an administrative function for their employees. Individual consumers and families will be encouraged to plan and finance the purchase of their health care services through their choice of self-insurance or conventional health insurance benefits. Either option will offer free choice of health care providers or, as the third option, participation in an integrated health care financing-delivery organization.

Health care providers will be encouraged to compete for consumers locally, either through continued participation in the fee-for-service market (but with much greater consumer sensitivity to fees); through participation in the comprehensive health care delivery organizations that are paid on a capitation basis; or through wholly new, innovative approaches that better meet consumers' health care wants. The advantage of paying for services with the consumer's own resources is that the consumer can choose the kind of services that are provided.

Instead of trying to constrain competitive market controls and consumer freedom of choice, as the managed competition proposals for health care reform do, this proposal seeks to prevent the past failures that inflicted the health care market—"free" first-dollar health insurance and incentives to insurers and employers to avoid insuring or employing high-risk persons. These provisions ultimately deprived consumers of their appropriate decision-making role in the health care market and led to provider domination of the market, however well-meaning their intentions. This market had no competitive coercion to "reduce prices, weed out inefficient producers, apply the spur of ruthless necessity to the others, all for the benefit of the public."

An appendix to the chapter contains a summary of the innovative competition approach to health care reform in a legislative format. Such legislation would meet the twin objectives of providing universal insurance coverage and correcting the flaws in the health care market that prevent the consumer from assuming the key role in making health care decisions. It utilizes the framework of the Clinton proposal with parts of the single-payer, the Cooper mandate, and the Jackson Hole approaches; and it could be drafted into a much shorter bill than 1,342 pages.

WHAT ELSE CAN BE GAINED FROM REFORM

Health care reform involves more than health care. It also affects government entitlements, job creation, balancing the federal budget, and more. As was noted in the introductory chapter, the auto and the computer industries served as the lighting rods for changes earlier in the nation's economic development. Today the health care industry is in that spotlight. By commanding one-seventh of the nation's resources, providing one-eleventh of all jobs, and being of central importance to all labor-management negotiations as the most prized and vigorously defended labor fringe benefit of 84 percent of all employed persons, the health care industry has an importance beyond its services for health.

Finally, restraining the extraordinarily high rate of increase in health care spending over the last four decades through health care reform will have a profound effect on the budgets of government at all levels, as well as the consumer's. "Even if we miraculously balanced the [federal] budget next year and kept every other program from growing at all, runaway medical bills alone would just about put us back where we started by the end of the decade" [Peterson, 1993]. The key to containing both overall health care costs and the government's share of those costs is to redefine the health entitlement in terms of universal coverage of unaffordable health care costs as determined by the relationship of those costs to family income. The government can no longer, if it ever could, afford to provide health services to those whose income is sufficient to provide these services for themselves. Providing free services to those who can afford to provide for themselves distorts specific markets and the general economy in ways that in an era of international competitiveness we can no longer afford.

Freeing business from the fixed costs of health care benefits per employee should make permanent job positions more attractive and labor negotiations over wages more straightforward and easier to relate to productivity changes. Fuchs [1993b] points out that:

> When health insurance was a small percentage of total compensation, and when most insurance premiums were community rated (not firm specific as at present), the distortions were small. Now they are becoming large. Today, workers' choice of job, decisions about job choices, and timing of retirement are frequently influenced by health insurance considerations. As a result, labor market efficiency suffers. It also suffers when, as is becoming more common, employers decisions about hiring, training, promotion, and firing are influenced by the impact of such decisions on health care costs.

The promise of a health care reform plan, designed to correct the flaws in the health care marketplace, is great. Not only will reform of the health care market make needed services available to all citizens on an equitable basis, but it will also extend the healing power of rational choice, based on real costs and personal assessment of benefit, to government fiscal managment and the labor market—enhancing job opportunities and preserving equity between labor and management. Government's role in the reformed health care system would be extended as the insurer of last resort to ensure equity in financing of and the availability of health services. However, the federal government would no longer need to distort health care markets by acting as a discriminating oligopsonist in the purchase of health services because of the dilemma of having to match unlimited entitlement commitments with a fixed budget constraint.

APPENDIX

THE AFFORDABLE HEALTH CARE REFORM, UNIVERSAL HEALTH INSURANCE, AND EMPLOYMENT REVITALIZATION ACT

Purposes

1. To initiate fundamental reform of the nation's health care financing and delivery system by:

   A. providing financial assistance by the federal government to all citizens and alien residents, in accordance with the person's ability to pay, for the purchase of health care services; and,

   B. containing health care costs through a restructuring of private health insurance to limit consumers' liability according to family income and to eliminate the risk of catastrophic illness from health insurance carriers and comprehensive health care delivery organizations.

2. To encourage the employment of additional full-time employees and to stimulate economic recovery by:

   A. limiting the employer's obligation for employees health insurance benefits to existing levels and reducing their obligations for retired employees health benefits; and,

   B. providing incentives for economic growth to American businesses by lowering fixed labor costs and reducing their retirement liabilities and to consumers by providing a portable set of building-block health care insurance benefits and, in the transition, making it possible to increase their aggregate net cash wages.

3. To accomplish the first two objectives without either increasing the national debt or risking the future of the nation's health care delivery system on a single, untried method of organizing and financing health care services by:

A. limiting the federal government's obligation for financing health care services to the aged and disabled, through an enriched Medicare program, and persons whose family income is below the poverty level or who are catastrophically ill and by raising tax revenues necessary for the full financing of program costs through means that are either progressive or will promote healthier life-styles; and,

B. requiring state administration of the program to ensure systematic experimentation with alternative methods of controlling and organizing health care delivery.

Health Care Benefits

1. The definition of health care services that will qualify for federal financial assistance are the benefits described in the Health Security Act with some modification of the deductibles and copayments according to family income. Persons who are aged 65 and over or are classified as permanently disabled at the time this act goes into operation shall continue to be eligible for Medicare benefits for the remainder of their lives.

2. The amount of direct federal financial assistance available to any individual will be determined by the individual's family income and the excess of expenditures for these comprehensive health care services made by the individual or family over a deductible of 5 percent of that family income plus copayments of 50 percent of an additional 10 percent of the family income for all citizens except lower-income families, who are defined as individuals whose family income is below the poverty level, and individuals entitled to Medicare benefits. The lower-income families, in lieu of Medicaid which shall be terminated by amendment of the Social Security Act, shall be eligible for federal financial assistance without any deductible or copayment and the Medicare beneficiaries shall be limited to a deductible, based only on their personal out-of-pocket expenditures, of 10 percent of family income.

3. In addition to direct federal assistance, the federal government will establish a loan guarantee program for assisting individuals in obtaining postcare financing through Health Care Financing Assistance Agencies for their out-of-pocket health care service costs. The federal government, through the Internal Revenue Service, will assist

the financing agencies in the collection of those obligations that become past due.

Financing Federal Program Costs

1. The primary source of financing the program costs will be through amendment of the Internal Revenue Code to redefine taxable income for individuals to include payments made by employers for health insurance premiums on the individual's behalf. [See the section on Program Transition for an employee option to convert employer health premiums into cash salaries.]

2. The secondary source of financing will be the same increases in the so-called "sin" taxes on tobacco that are included in the Health Security Act.

3. During the first five years of the program's operation, a third source of financing will be payments from state governments in amounts initially equal to their Medicaid expenditures in the year prior to program implementation. These payments will decline by at least 20 percent in each of the first five years of the program and the rate of decline may increase even more rapidly if the National Health Board concludes that a particular state's performance in meeting its responsibilities for administering the federal program produces superior reduction in the state's rate of health care inflation.

Program Administration

1. Overall direction for the administration of the program will be the responsibility of the National Health Board similar to the body included in the Health Security Act except that this body will be limited to overseeing and evaluating the program and monitoring the state program performance; approving different types of state experiments with health care financing and regulation; and periodically reporting on the health insurance programs operation to the Congress and recommending legislative changes.

2. Each state would be required to establish an authority for administering the federal program in accordance with federal standards established in the legislation. In addition to ensuring that each U.S. citizen and resident alien receives the catastrophic health insurance benefits and that HMO registration for low-income beneficiaries is competitively bid and low-income beneficiaries are assigned to con-

venient and accessable HMOs, these standards include a plan for expanding primary care in the state, a plan for the management of care for the catastrophically ill, and a program for approving and monitoring Health Care Financing Assistance Agencies that ensure that each citizen has a choice of agencies for receiving all his/her benefits from the federal assistance program and certifies the agency's competence to provide other financing or health services. If the state cannot develop a satisfactory plan or subsequently does not make sufficient progress in accomplishing its goals, then the federal government would be required to administer an appropriate plan for that state.

3. Health Care Financing Assistance Agencies will be responsible for ensuring that all residents receive their benefits for federal assistance, arranging post-care loans for obligations citizens incur in purchasing qualified health services, and can offer other services as certified by the state health agency to assist residents with the financing and consumption of health care services.

Program Operation and Transition

1. In the year of implementation each employee receiving employer-purchased health insurance would have the option of either directing the employer to pay an amount equal to all or part of the previous year's premium to his/her designated Health Care Financing Assistance Agency, or to have the employer increase his/her wages by all or part of that last year's premium. However, the employer's future obligation for employee health benefits would be fixed at whatever dollar amount the employee designates in the year of implementation unless the employer agrees to increase the contribution in future wage negotiations. All employers are, however, obligated to make available to all employees the opportunity to purchase health insurance and offer several insurance options as defined by the National Health Board.

2. The legislation would include a plan detailing the time schedule for establishing the National Health Board, the development and approval of the state health plans, the mechanism for exercising the individual's choice of Health Care Financing Assistance Agency and the employee's direction to his/her employer of either premium designation or increased cash wages.

Chapter Notes

CHAPTER 2

1. Flexner, said to be the most influential layman in American medical history, was a liberal arts graduate of Johns Hopkins, and his physician brother was the long-time director of the Rockefeller Foundation. According to Flexner's report there were some 22,000 medical and osteopathic students in training during 1906–1909, when his medical school surveys were conducted. Harvard, Johns Hopkins, and Western Reserve, which were the only three schools fully qualified for medical education in his view, had only 680 students enrolled. Another 3,371 students were enrolled in programs that required at least some college work for admission to medical school. Thus, less than 20 percent of the medical students were enrolled in programs that had realistic admission standards.

2. In urban areas, especially at the most prestigious institutions, the specialists captured control of the medical staff positions, and the closed-staff model became dominant in most urban hospitals. Corwin [1946, 45–46] reported that less than 30 percent of the physicians in Cleveland had hospital medical staff appointments and that slightly more than 33 percent of the physicians in New York City in 1921 had hospital affiliations. The vast majority of those physicians with medical staff appointments, in New York at least, had privileges in only one hospital. Because the specialists were concentrated in the major cities and towns [Stevens 1971, 180–181], a different, more open style of hospital medical staffing developed in the hinterlands where 48 percent of all Americans lived in 1929. However, only 30 percent of the physicians practiced in rural areas. Whereas "in 1929 there were 126 physicians for each 100,000 of the population in the United States, the concentration ranged from as low as 78 per 100,000 in all towns of 5,000 or less to an average of 180 in all towns of 1,000,000,000 and over, or approximately 185 for all town of 100,000 or over" [Falk et al 1928, 197–198]. The distribution of physicians and

hospital beds were even more skewed toward urban areas where higher income citizens resided; e.g., Falk et al [1928] found that "the concentration of physicians is almost in direct proportion to the estimated per-capita wealth of the location in which they had settled."

3. During this era and until his retirement in 1949, the American Medical Association's public policies were dominated by one man, Morris Fishbein, M.D., who was the editor of the *Journal of the American Medical Association* (JAMA). Fishbein was responsible for the outspoken attack on the CCMC report, describing it as a tool of "the great foundations, public health official-dom, social theory—even socialism and communism—inciting to revolution," even though the committee's chairman, Ray Lyman Wilbur, was a past president of the AMA. He opposed voluntary as well as public health insurance and closed panel group practice or, as he described it, "contract medicine." When in 1938 the Justice Department obtained criminal indictments against the AMA and four other medical societies for antitrust violations in denying hospital privileges to physicians associated with the Group Health Association of Washington, Fishbein was one of the 21 individuals also indicted. In addition to his strong personality and enormous experience, the advertising in Fishbein's journal was responsible for virtually all of the AMA's revenues; doctors did not pay dues to belong to the AMA until after his retirement. Fishbein's public statements may have been more vitriolic than the views of organized medicine, but they certainly were consistent with the mainstream medical practitioner, and the AMA took a long time after Fishbein's retirement to embrace group practice and what later became the HMO [Campion, 1984].

4. Although the idea of Blue Cross has often been associated with the Baylor plan, the cooperative rather than competitive nature of the arrangement is more like the consumer associations in the midwest that had been established much earlier. For example, in 1912 a cooperative hospital prepayment program had been organized in Rockford, Illinois, in which "any resident of the community is eligible to membership provided he is over 15 years of age and is free from chronic illness and from all physical defects requiring hospitalization" [Falk et al 1928, 478]. For an entrance fee and small weekly contributions, the member was entitled to six weeks hospitalization a year in any local hospital, a fixed allowance for operating room fees, and some services of a visiting nurse for non-hospitalized illnesses. A similar program existed in Grinnell, Iowa, during the 1920s and another was organized in Brattleboro, Vermont, in 1927. These prepayment programs were organized by consumers independent of health care providers. The only difference between these cooperatives and Blue Cross was that hospitals rather than consumers formed the cooperative; i.e., it was a producer cooperative.

CHAPTER 3

5. A major exception to the lack of change during the wartime period was the federal government's first effort to purchase health care from the private sector. The Emergency Maternity and Infant Care Program was estab-

lished in 1943 to provide care for wives and dependents of servicemen. Although the program lasted only four years, it established two precedents that influenced the development of subsequent federal programs for purchasing health care services from private providers. First, cost was established as the basis for pricing hospital services [Wolkstein 1968]. Second, the program, directed by the Children's Bureau, employed cooperative arrangements with state health departments for its administration [Anderson 1968, 116–117].

6. The acceleration of federal government activity in health care can be seen from the pace of congressional legislation. As part of the nation's bicentennial celebration, the Department of Health, Education, and Welfare [1976] prepared a chronology of major federal health legislation enacted since the ratification of the U.S. Constitution in 1788 until the bicentennial in 1976. Of the 170 pieces of health-related legislation identified by HEW staff, only 46 specific pieces of legislation were enacted prior to 1940. Nearly three-fourths were approved after 1940 with exactly 50 percent coming after 1960.

The federal government's involvement in health issues had been minimal prior to 1941. Nevertheless, during the 150 years from 1789 to 1940, every possible form of government intervention into private markets had been tried, at least in limited form, except antitrust enforcement or direct economic regulation of the health care industry.

The most extreme form of intervention in health care is for the government to impose new taxes and provide a uniform set of health care benefits for everyone. In a limited way, the Fifth Congress in 1798 enacted such a program. The Act for the Relief of Sick and Disabled Seamen imposed a tax on a seamen's wages and established a governmentally owned and operated health care delivery system (true socialism), the Merchant Marine Hospitals. This nation's first and only compulsory health insurance program continued until 1884 when the tax on seamen's wages was abolished. However, the governmental health service for the merchant marine lasted until the Reagan Administration's dismantling of the Public Health Service hospitals.

In addition to governmentally-operated health services to the merchant marine and to members of the U.S. military, legislation was enacted to establish federal Old Soldiers Homes in 1866 after the Civil War and the Veterans Administration in 1921 after World War I. This approach differs from federal programs to purchase medical services from private physicians and hospitals, as had been done in both of those wars. This practice was continued in 1922 with the Sheppard-Towner Act, which supported maternal and child welfare programs and aided blind and crippled children until it was rescinded in 1929. These benefits were restored in Title V of the Social Security Act in 1935 and fully reinstated for dependents of servicemen in the direct purchase of medical services through the Emergency Maternity and Infant Care program from 1943 to 1947.

However, the most urgent reason for government to intervene in the operation of private markets is to protect the health and safety of its citizens through the promulgation of rules and regulations governing private behavior in both the marketplace and personal life. Congressional legislative initiatives in the 1790s and early 1800s concerned the federal government's authority to issue health and safety regulations. In this period Congress limited the scope of federal health and safety regulation to maritime activities, such as quarantine regulations in American ports of entry. Congress drew upon the U.S. government's authority to regulate foreign commerce as the basis for the federal health and safety regulatory program. Nevertheless, state governments were seen as the primary protectors of health and safety.

State governmental jurisdiction over public health prevailed until Congress finally accepted responsibility for federal regulation of interstate commerce in the railroad industry in 1887. Federal health and safety legislation proliferated in the 1890s and throughout the progressive era. These programs encompassed interstate quarantine laws; control of waste dumping in navigable waters; licensing and regulation of the sale of serums and vaccines; regular inspection of meat packing plants; prohibition of misbranded or adulterated food, drinks, or drugs; a similar prohibition on insecticides; prohibition of false and misleading therapeutic claims in the labeling of medicines; and federal controls over narcotics users and suppliers.

In 1902 the United States Public Health Service was established to replace the Marine Hospital Service and to expand the corps of civil servants with medical and health care expertise to carry out the federal government's growing responsibilities in health and safety regulation, to care for maritime seamen, and to conduct research on infectious diseases and other public health problems. Even with this expansion of federal regulatory authority, the predominant control of health and safety regulation remained at the state level. Except for the manufacture and sale of drugs, state control of physicians, other health care personnel, and hospital licensure to protect patients remained as the primary instrument of regulation in the private health care market.

7. In the history of health care there have been many allegations of conspiratorial conduct. For example, E. Richard Brown [1979a] documents the role foundations (capitalists) played in shaping the conspiracy of scientific medicine to control medical education at the turn of the century; Sylvia A. Law [1974] argues that Blue Cross was primarily accountable to hospitals, not the general public; and Paul Starr [1982b], in the most complex thesis, portrays organized medicine's activities as a single-minded effort to achieve cultural authority and, thus, professional dominance for increased social and economic power. However, few conspiracies in health care are as well documented and open as the Lasker cabal. Advocates of basic science in medical education and the profession were the primary beneficiaries without their active involvement.

CHAPTER 4

8. William Kissick recently expressed the view that Wilbur Cohn, who in 1965 was the assistant secretary for legislation in the Department of Health Education, and Welfare, "wrote Medicare and worked very closely with . . . [Congressman Mills] to get the legislation passed and then made certain that Wilbur Mills got credit for it" [Murata 1993]. Cohn, a career public servant,

came to Washington as part of the Roosevelt brain trust in the '30s and participated in the drafting of the original Social Security Act of 1935. He became HEW Secretary later in the Johnson Administration to cap a very distinguished career in the social welfare field. His contributions to the drafting and the successful implementation of the Medicare program were indeed very significant.

9. The SSA had selected a method of apportioning costs to Medicare patients that reduced program costs substantially below the average cost per diem method of apportionment that was used by most Blue Cross plans and had been employed in previous federal programs. As a final accommodation to the providers a 2 percent allowance in lieu of specific costs, the "plus factor," was added to the reimbursement formula. It proved to be so controversial that hearings were held by the Senate Finance Committee to review its legitimacy in light of the statutory requirement that hospitals should be paid their "reasonable costs" for caring for Medicare patients. The Government Accounting Office found that "there is sufficient merit to the concepts involved when viewed in the context of the statutory provision authorizing the use of estimates to preclude our concluding that the allowance in question is illegal." Because of GAO's ringing endorsement, the committee, with an 11 to 6 Democratic majority, ratified the reimbursement formula with what Senator Paul Douglas of Illinois described as "sweeteners or grease" to prime the program pump.

Hospitals felt very strongly about the plus factor. When the Nixon Administration removed it in 1969 they created such a stir in Washington that the new administration had to add an 8.5 percent nursing factor to the reimbursement formula to restore equity in apportionment and give hospitals back about one-half of the dollars lost in the elimination of the plus factor.

10. The 89th Congress did not stop with PL 89–97. It went on to pass more significant health legislation than any other two-year session in the history of the U.S. Congress. It passed the Heart Disease, Cancer, and Stroke Amendments (PL 89–239), which established Regional Medical Programs for research training and sharing of new knowledge about these diseases; the Comprehensive Health Planning and Public Health Services Amendments (PL 89–749), which promoted health planning and improved public health services and authorized broad research, demonstration, and training programs in federal-state-local partnerships; the initial legislation requiring warning labels on cigarettes; several environmental measures, such as amendments to the Clean Air Act and Clean Water Restoration Act, and enacted the National Traffic and Motor Vehicle Safety Act; the original school breakfast program as a part of the Child Nutrition Act; and the initial effort to support training of allied health workers and a loan program for health professionals.

11. The Robinson-Luft study began in 1972, but its findings reflect increases in hospital personnel and investments in plant assets that occurred after 1966. Pettengil [1973] reports a marked increase in the number of hospital personnel (more than doubling) and plant assets (more than 50 percent higher) per 100 census over the levels in the five years before Medicare-Medicaid.

12. Davis et al [1987] catalog the significant mortality gains that have been made by black Americans since 1960. Davis credits both programs with permitting minority and low-income groups to share in the major health gains.

13. The term "health maintenance organization" or HMO was coined by Paul M. Ellwood, Jr., and referred to comprehensive health care delivery organizations that would be paid through annual capitation fees. Ellwood believed that the capitation payment would provide an incentive for the organization to keep its enrollees well rather than be encouraged to find and treat as much illness as possible [Falkson, 1980].

14. One indication of the success of the for-profit public relations campaign and the chain movement being viewed as a threat to the rest of the industry was the appointment of the Committee on Implications of For-Profit Enterprise in Health Care by the Institute of Medicine in 1983 to study investor-owned chains of health care facilities. The committee reported that the investor-owned systems did not possess management that was superior to the management of not-for-profit hospitals. By comparing similar not-for-profit and for-profit hospitals, it concluded that for-profit chain hospitals "have slightly higher expenses than not-for-profit institutions, charge more per stay, have achieved higher levels of profitability before and after taxes, and respond more precisely to economic incentives." Neither superior economic performance nor better cost restraint was exhibited by the for-profits. As for quality of care, the committee concluded that "investor-owned hospitals are similar in quality to not-for-profit hospitals, and on some measures they are better." Evidently, providing and documenting high quality of care in their hospitals was good business. The report's most important conclusion did not even pertain to investor-owned hospitals, but rather to the effect of profit-seeking behavior on the fiduciary responsibilies of physicians—a topic to be taken up in the next chapter.

15. As a consequence of the substantial program cost overruns, the tax provisions for financing the hospital program had to be amended frequently. From the original payroll tax with a combined rate of 1 percent for the first full year of Medicare (1967) on earnings up to $7,800 with scheduled increases to occur gradually in both the rate and the earnings base, the combined rate had reached 3.3 percent and in 1993 the base finally was made applicable to all earned wages.

CHAPTER 5

16. Even at this much lower level of occupancy, the hospital industry still utilized its capital facilities at level comparable to the nation's hotel industry, which had an occupancy ratio of 61.7 percent in 1992 [McDowell 1993]. The economic efficiency of the hospital is more sensitive to the level of staffing than to the occupancy level unless the facilities have been financed principally with debt.

17. In 1992 300 multihospital systems owned, controlled, or managed 2,826 hospitals with 540,099 beds, 43.2 percent of all hospitals and 45.8 percent of total (both long and short-term) beds [AHA *Guide* and *Hospital Statistics*, 1993].

18. This respite in the rate of hospital inflation was not reflected in Medicare program expenditures, which contined to rise at 20.6 and 17.1 percent in 1982 and 1983, because the elderly's rate of admissions continued to increase while the under 65 rate fell. Thus, the Medicare program should have had a larger apportionment of total hospital costs allocated to it in addition to the double-digit average rate of increase in other health care costs.

19. The DRGs were developed by two professors, R.B. Fetter and J.D. Thompson, at Yale University's Institute for Social and Policy Studies in the early 1970s as a tool for patient care evaluation. However, because the diagnostic groupings were based on the relative level of resources that should be required to care for patients with particular admitting diagnoses, this patient classification scheme was also used for planning and budgeting. By the relative weighting of resource requirements for various groups of diagnoses, the methodology provided a convenient means of allocating costs within the hospital and establishing prices for each of the admitting diagnoses. The method was field tested in the late '70s in Connecticut, New Jersey, and Pennsylvaia and then employed in a reimbursement experiment with New Jersey hospitals beginning in 1979 and continuing into the early 1980s.

20. Since 1963 when the National Hospital Panel Survey was established, hospitals had until 1979 reported small negative operating margins from patient activities, i.e., patient revenues were less than total expenses. However, revenues from nonpatient care activities have been large enough on average to earn a postive total operating margin for the average hospital of 2 or 3 percent in the 1960s and '70s and 4 or 5 percent of total revenues in the 1980s and 90s. In the first two years of Medicare PPS both patient margins, 2 and 1.5 percent respectively. and total operating margins, 6.2 and 5.9 percent, were at record levels in 1984 and 1985.

21. Physician services are defined as the categories of direct expenses of physicians and of other professional services because the latter services include outpatient clinics and dialysis centers.

CHAPTER 7

22. The "Jackson Hole Group" is a discussion group of 33 persons knowledgable and interested in health policy and reform. The group was organized by Paul M. Ellwood, M.D., president of InterStudy and the father of the HMO concept, and Alain C. Enthoven, Ph.D., who is a professor in Stanford University's Graduate School of Business and the author of *Health Plan, The Only Practical Solution to the Soaring Cost of Medical Care*. It was named for the location, Jackson Hole, Wyoming, of its meetings.

23. As reported in chapter 6, the aged consumed 36.3 percent of the nation's health care spending in 1987, and their relative share of spending had been growing at nearly 2 percent per annum over the previous decade.

24. A Foster Higgins and Co. survey on 1991 employer premiums ranging from $2,891 in the wholesale/retail industry to more than $4,500 in the utility industry, with a median between $3,479 and $3,861.

25. Although the use of nurse practitioners to provide primary care services will continue to be a responsibility of state licensing agencies, consumer acceptance through a market test will play a more significant role in determining the success of this change. Currently, the delivery organization captures most of savings arising from the substitution of nurse practitioners for physicians, but in a reformed market consumers, as well as the nurses, would realize the benefits from the lower health care costs.

26. The federal government's track record for collecting sums owed it has not been outstanding—except for the Internal Revenue Service. Therefore, it is proposed that any past-due sums owed the federal government as part of the citizen's postcare loan program become collectible by IRS.

References

American Hospital Association (AHA). *Hospitals, Journal of AHA*, August 1, Part II, various years from 1945 to 1972, and *AHA Hospital Statistics*, various years after 1972.

————. 1977. *Hospital Regulation, Report of the Special Committee on the Regulatory Process*. Chicago: AHA.

————. 1981. *Data Book on Multi-Hospital Systems*. Chicago: AHA.

————. 1992. *Ambulatory Care Trendlines, 1992*. Chicago: AHA.

————. 1993. *The Guide to the Health Care Field*. Chicago: AHA.

American Medical Association (AMA). 1968. *Survey of Medical Groups in the U.S., 1965*. Chicago: AMA.

Andersen, Ronald, Smedby, Bjorn, and Anderson, Odin W. 1968. *Medical Care Use in Sweden and the United States—A Comparative Analysis of Systems and Behavior*, Chicago: Center for Health Administration Studies, University of Chicago.

Anderson, Odin W. 1968. *The Uneasy Equilibrium: Private and Public Financing of Health Services in the United States, 1875–1965*. New Haven, CT: College and University Press.

————. 1975. *Blue Cross Since 1929: Accountability and the Public Trust*. Cambridge, MA: Ballinger Publishing Co.

————. 1985. *Health Services in the United States: A Growth Enterprise Since 1875*. Ann Arbor, MI: Health Administration Press.

Barlett, Donald C., and Steele, James B. 1992. *America: What Went Wrong*. Kansas City, MO: Andrews and McMeel.

Baumol, William. 1993. "Health Reform Can't Cure High Costs." *New York Times*. August 8.

Becker, Harry, ed. 1955. *Prepayment and the Community: Financing Hospital Care in the United States*, vol 2. New York: McGaw-Hill Book Company, Inc.

Belloc, Nedra B., and Breslow, Lester. 1972. "Relationship of Physical Health Status and Health Practices." *Preventive Medicine*. 1: 409–21.

Berk, Marc L., and Monheit, Alan C. 1992. "The Concentration of Health Expenditures: An Update." *Health Affairs*. 11: (Winter) 145–149.

Birnbaum, Jeffrey H., and Murray, Alan S. 1987. *Showdown at Gucci Gulch, Lawmakers, Lobbyists, and the Unlikely Triumph of Tax Reform*. New York: Random House.

Blendon, Robert J., and Donelan, Karen. 1990. "The Public and the Emerging Debate over National Health Insurance." *New England Journal of Medicine*. 323: (July 19) 208–212.

Bloom, Gordon F., and Northrup, Herbert R. 1955. *Economics of Labor Relations*. Homewood, IL: Richard D. Irwin, Inc.

Breslow, Lester. 1978. "Risk Factor Intervention for Health Maintenance." *Science*. 200: 908–912.

Brooks, Robert H., Ware, John E., Jr., Rodgers, William H., Keeler, Emmett B., Davies, Allyson R., Donald, Cathy A., Goldberg, George A., Lohr, Kathleen N., Masthay, Patricia C., and Newhouse, Joseph P. 1983. "Does Free Care Improve Adults' Health? Results from a Randomized Controlled Trial." *New England Journal of Medicine*. 309: (Dec 8) 1426–1434.

Brown, E. Richard. 1979a. *Rockefeller Medicine Men: Medicine and Capitalism in America*. Berkeley and Los Angeles: University of California Press.

———. 1979b. "He Who Pays the Piper: Foundations, the Medical Profession, and Medical Education." In *Health Care in America, Essays in Social History*. Reverby, Susan, and Rosner, David, ed. Philadelphia: Temple University Press.

Bugbee, George. 1959. "The Physician in the Hospital Organization." *New England Journal of Medicine*. 261: (Oct. 29) 896–901.

Burnstein, Helen R., Lipsitz, Stuart R., and Brennan, Troyen A. 1992. "Socioeconomic Status and Risk for Substandard Care." *Journal of the American Medical Association*. 268: (November 4) 2383–2387.

Campion, Frank D. 1984. *The AMA and U.S. Health Policy Since 1940*. Chicago: Chicago Review Press.

Carpenter, Theodore M. 1994. "Opportunities to Create Networks Now." In *Creating Community Care Net-works: Issues and Opportunities, Report of the 1993 National Forum on Hospital and Health Affairs*. J. Alexander McMahon, ed. Durham, NC: Fuqua School of Business, Duke University.

Chandler, Alfred D., Jr. 1977. *The Visible Hand, The Management Revolution in American Business*. Cambridge: Belknap Press of Harvard University Press.

Clapesattle, Helen B. 1954. *The Doctors Mayo*. Minneapolis: University of Minnesota Press.

Clark, J.M. 1939. *Social Control of Business*. New York: McGraw-Hill Book Company.

Clymer, Adam. 1993. "Clinton Asks Backing for Sweeping Change in the Health System." *New York Times*. September 23.

Committee on the Costs of Medical Care. 1932. *Medical Care for the American People: The Final Report of the Committee on the Costs of Medical Care.* Chicago: University of Chicago Press.

Cooper, Philip F., and Monheit, Alan C. 1993. "Does Employment-Related Health Insurance Inhibit Job Mobility?" *Inquiry.* 30: (Winter) 400–416.

Corning, Peter A. 1969. *The Evolution of Medicare . . . from idea to law.* Washington, DC: U.S.Department of Health, Education, and Welfare.

Corwin, E. H. L. 1924. *The Hospital Situation in Greater New York, Report of a Survey of Hospitals in New York City by the Public Health Committee of the New York Academy of Medicine.* New York: G. P. Putnam's Sons.

———. 1946. *The American Hospital.* New York: The Commonwealth Fund.

Council of Economic Advisers. 1993. *Economic Report of the President.* Washington, DC: United States Government Printing Office.

Davis, Karen; Lillie-Blanton, Marsha; Lyons, Barbara; Mullan, Fitzhugh; Powe, Neil; and Rowland, Diane. 1987. "Health Care for Black Americans: The Public Sector Role." *The Milbank Quarterly.* 65: (Suppl. 1) 213–247.

Davis, Michael M. 1955. *Medical Care for Tomorrow.* New York: Harper & Brothers Publishers.

Delano, Barbara G., Feinroth, Mary V., Feinroth, Martin, and Friedman, Eli A. 1981. "Home and Medical Center Hemodialysis—Dollar Comparison and Payback Period." *Journal of American Medical Association.* 246: (July 17) 230–232.

Drake, David F. 1978. "Does Money Spent on Health Care Really Improve U.S. Health Status?" *Hospitals.* 52: (October, 16) 63–65.

———. 1980 "The Cost of Hospital Regulation." Arthur Levin, ed. *Regulating Health Care: The Struggle for Control.* New York: Academy of Political Science.

Drake, David F., and Raske, Kenneth E. 1974. "The Changing Hospital Economy." *Hospitals.* 48: (November 16) 34–40.

Eilers, Robert D., and Moyerman, Sue S., ed. 1971. *National Health Insurance, Proceedings of the Conference on National Health Insurance.* Homewood, IL: Richard D. Irwin, Inc. for the Leonard Davis Institute of Health Economics.

Eisenberg, Howard. 1980. "'Convenience Clinics' Your Newest Rival for Patients?" *Medical Economics.* 57: (November 24) 71–75, 79,81, and 84.

Ellwood, Paul M., Enthoven, Alain C., and Etheredge, Lynn M. 1992. "The Jackson Hole Initiatives for a Twenty-First Century American Health System." *Health Economics.* 1: 149–168.

Enthoven, Alain C. 1980. *Health Plan, The Only Practical Solution to the Soaring Cost of Medical Care.* Reading MA: Addison-Wesley Publishing Co.

———. 1993. "Why Managed Care Has Failed to Contain Health Care Costs." *Health Affairs.* 12: (Fall) 27–43.

Falk, I. S., Rorem, C. Rufus, and Ring, Martha D. 1933. *The Costs of Medical Care: A Summary.* Committee on the Costs of Medical Care Publication No. 27. Chicago: University of Chicago Press.

Falkson, Joseph L. 1980. *HMOs and the Politics of Health System Reform*. Chicago: American Hospital Association.

Fein, Rashi. 1967. *The Doctor Shortage: An Economic Diagnosis*, Washington, DC: Brookings Institution.

Feldman, Roger. 1993. "Who Pays for Mandated Health Insurance Benefits?" *Journal of Health Economics*. 11: 341–348.

Feldstein, Martin S. 1971. *The Rising Cost of Hospital Care*, Washington, DC: Information Resources Press.

Feldstein, Martin S., and Taylor, Amy K. 1977. *The Rapid Rise of Hospital Costs*. Washington, DC: Executive Office of the President.

Feldstein, Paul J. 1979. *Health Care Economics*. New York: John Wiley & Sons.

Fisher, Charles R. 1980. "Differences by Age Groups in Health Care Spending." *Health Care Financing Review*. 1: (Spring) 65–90.

Fleming, Scott. 1971. "Anatomy of the Kaiser-Permanente Program," Anne R. Somers, ed. *The Kaiser-Permanente Medical Care Program*. New York: The Commonwealth Fund.

Flexner, Abraham. 1910. *Medical Education in the United States and Canada, A Report to Carnegie Foundation for the Advancement of Teaching*. New York: Carnegie Foundation.

Foster, Richard W. 1976. "The Financial Structure of Community Hospitals: Impact of Medicare. In *The Nature of Hospital Costs: Three Studies*. Chicago: Hospital Research and Education Trust.

Freshnock, Larry J., and Jensen, Lynn E. 1981. "The Changing Structure of Medical Group Practice in the United States, 1969 to 1980." *Journal of American Medical Association*. 245: (June 5) 2173–2176.

Freymann, John Gordon. 1974. *The American Health Care System: Its Genesis and Trajectory*. New York: Medicom Press.

Fuchs, Victor R. 1969. "What Kind of System for Health Care?" *Bulletin of the New York Academy of Medicine*. 45: (March) 281–292.

———. 1979. "The Economics of Health in a Post-Industrial Society." *Public Interest*. 56: (Summer) 3–20.

———. 1993a. "No Pain, No Gain—Perspectives on Cost Containment." *Journal of American Medical Association*. 269: (Feb 3) 631–633.

———. 1993b. *The Future of Health Policy*. Cambridge, MA: Harvard University Press.

Fuchs, Victor R., and Hahn, James S. 1990. "A Comparison of Expenditures for Physicians' Services in the United States and Canada." *New England Journal of Medicine*. 323: (Sept. 27) 884–890.

Gearon, Christopher J. 1994. "Employer Mandate, Will it survive the battle?" *AHA News*. 30: (January 10).

Gibson, Robert M., Waldo, Daniel R., and Levit, Katharine R. 1983. "National Health Expenditures, 1982." *Health Care Financing Review*. 5: (Fall) 1–31.

Goldberg, Lawrence G. and Greenberg, Warren. 1978. "The Emergence of Physician-Sponsored Health Insurance: A Historical Perspective." Greenberg, Warren ed. *Competition in the Health Care Sector: Past, Present, and Future*. Washington, DC: Federal Trade Commission.

Goldfarb, David L., Mintz, Ruth, and Yeager, Martin S. 1982. "Why Did Hospital Costs Increase in 1981?" *Hospitals*. 56: (July 15) 109–114.

Gregg, Alan. 1956. *Challenges to Contemporary Medicine*. New York: Columbia University Press.

Harris, Richard. 1966. "Annuals of Legislation: Medicare (4 parts)." *New Yorker*. July 2, 9, 16, and 23, and subsequently published as *A Sacred Trust*, New York: New American Library, Inc.

Henderson, John. 1991. "Surgery centers continue pattern of growth." *Modern Healthcare*. 21: (June 3) 36–37.

Hiatt, Howard H. 1991. "Meet Dr. Jarman. He Makes House Calls." *New York Times*. November 16.

Hollingsworth, J. Rogers; Hage, Jerald; and Hanneman, Robert A. 1990. *State Intervention in Medical Care: Consequences for Britain, France, Sweden, and the United States, 1890–1970*. Ithaca, NY: Cornell University Press.

Hsiao, William C., Dunn, Daniel L., and Verrilli, Diana K. 1993. "Assessing the Implementation of Physician-Payment Reform." *New England Journal of Medicine*. 328: (April 1) 928–933.

Iglehart, John K. 1982. "Funding the End-Stage Renal-Disease Program." *New England Journal of Medicine*. 306: (Feb 25) 492–496.

———. 1992. "The American Health Care System, Private Insurance." *New England Journal of Medicine*. 326: (June 18) 1715–1720.

———. 1993. "The American Health Care System, The End Stage Renal Disease Program." *New England Journal of Medicine*. 328: (Feb. 4) 366–371.

Ikegami, Naoki. 1991. "Japanese Health Care: Lower Cost through Regulated Fees." *Health Affairs*. 10: (Fall) 87–109.

Institute of Medicine Committee on Implications of For-Profit Enterprises in Health Care. 1986. *For-Profit Enterprise in Health Care*. Washington, DC: National Academy Press.

Kenkel, Paul J. 1993. "Kaiser Planning to Boost Point-of-Service Options." *Modern Healthcare*. 23: (September 20) 38.

Kessel, Reuben. 1958. "Price Discrimination in Medicine." *Journal of Law and Economics* 1: (October) 20–53.

King, Lester S. 1983a. "Clinical Science Gets Enthroned," Parts I and II. *Journal of American Medical Association*. 250: (September 2) 1169–1172 and (October 14) 1847–1850.

———. 1983b. "Medical Education: Elitisms and Reform." *Journal of American Medical Association*. 250: (November 11) 2457–2467.

———. 1984. "The Flexner Report of 1910." *Journal of American Medical Association*. 251: (February 24) 1079–1086.

Kingsdale, Jon Michael. 1981. *The Growth of Hospitals: An Economic History in Baltimore*. Unpublished doctoral dissertation. Ann Arbor: University of Michigan.

Kovar, Mary Grace. 1977. "Elderly People: The Population 65 Years and Over." *Health, United States, 1976–1977*. Washington, DC: U.S. Government Printing Office.

Kosterlitz, Julie. 1992a. "A Sick System." *National Journal*. 24: (February 15) 376–388.

———. 1992b. "Wanted: GPs." *National Journal*. 24: (September 5) 2011–2015.

———. 1992c. "We have met the future: Managed Care." *National Journal*. 24: (October 31) 2515.

Lave, Judith R. and Lave, Lester B. 1974. *The Hospital Construction Act: An Evaluation of the Hill-Burton Program, 1948–1983*. Washington, DC: American Enterprise Institute for Public Policy Research.

Law, Sylvia A. 1974. *Blue Cross: What Went Wrong?* New Haven: Yale University Press, Ltd.

Letsch, Suzanne W., Lazenby, Helen C., Levit, Katharine R., and Cowan, Cathy A. 1992. "National Health Expenditures, 1991." *Health Care Financing Review*. 14: (Winter) 1–30.

Levit, Katharine R., Lazenby, Helen, Waldo, Daniel R., and Davidoff, Lawrence M. 1985. "National Health Expenditures, 1984." *Health Care Financing Review*. 7: (Fall) 1–36.

Levit, Katharine R., Lazenby, Helen C., Cowan, Cathy A., and Letsch, Suzanne W. 1991. "National Health Expenditures, 1990." *Health Care Financing Review*. 13: (Fall) 29–54.

Levit, Katharine R, Olin, Gary L., and Letsch, Suzanne W. 1992. "Americans' health insurance coverage, 1980–91." *Health Care Financing Review*. 14: (Fall 1992) 31–57.

Leuchtenbury, William E. 1983. *In the Shadow of FDR, From Harry Truman to Ronald Reagan*. Ithaca, NY: Cornell University Press.

Levinsky, Norman G. 1993. "The Organization of Medical Care, Lessons from the Medicare End Stage Renal Disease Program." *New England Journal of Medicine*. 329: (November 4) 1395–1399.

Lovinger, Gail M. 1985. *AHA Policy Perspectives on Market Reform and Regulation in the Hospital Field, 1967–1984*. Chicago: AHA.

Luft, Harold S., and Miller, Robert H. 1988. "Patient Selection in a Competitive Health System." *Health Affairs*. 7: (Summer) 97–119.

MacIntyre, Duncan M. 1962. *Voluntary Health Insurance and Rate Making*. Ithaca, NY: Cornell University Press.

Mangan, Doreen. 1993. "How doctors are bailing out of self-referral facilities." *Medical Economics*. 70: (February 8) 182–188.

Markowitz, Gerald E., and Rosner, David. 1979. "Doctors in Crisis: Medical Education and Medical Reform During the Progressive Era, 1895–1915." In *Health Care in America: Essays in Social History*. Reverby, Susan and Rosner, David ed. Philadelphia: Temple University Press.

McConnel, Charles E., and Tobias, Lori A. 1986. "Distributional Change in Physician Manpower, United States, 1963–80." *Journal of American Public Health Association*. 76: (June) 638–642.

McDowell, Edwin. 1993. "Hotel Occupancy Rate Rises, New Figures Show." *New York Times*. (February 9).

McMahon, John Alexander, and Drake, David F. 1978. "Hospital Cost Containment: The American Hospital Association Perspective." Zubkoff,

Michael, Raskin, Ira E., and Hanft, Ruth S., ed. *Hospital Cost Containment: Selected Notes for Future Policy.* New York: PRODIST for the Milbank Memorial Fund.

Mechanic, David. 1978. *Medical Sociology* (2d ed.). New York: The Free Press.

Mitchell, Jean M. and Scott, Elton. 1992. "Physician Ownership of Physical Therapy Services." *Journal of American Medical Association.* 268: (October 21) 2055–2059.

Mitchell, Jean M., and Sunshine, Jonathan H. 1992. "Consequences of Physicians' Ownership of Health Care Facilities—Joint Ventures in Radiation Therapy." *New England Journal of Medicine.* 327: (November 19) 1497–1501.

Moloney, Thomas W., and Rogers, David E. 1979. "Medical Technology—A Different View of the Contentious Debate over Costs." *New England Journal of Medicine.* 304: (December 27) 1413–1419.

Morin, Richard, and Broder, David S. 1993. "Health Plan Doubts Abound." *Washington Post.* October 12.

Murata, Steve. 1993. "What lessons should we take from Medicare?" *Medical Economics.* 70: (June 28) 60–68.

National Centers for Health Statistics and Health Services Research. 1977. *Health, United States, 1976–1977.* Washington, DC: U.S. Department of Health, Education, and Welfare.

Neikirk, William. 1993. "Managed care may well mean less care." *Chicago Tribune.* December 6.

Office of National Cost Estimates. 1990. "National Health Expenditures, 1988." *Health Care Financing Review.* 11: (Summer) 1–41.

Pauly, Mark V. 1980. *Doctors and Their Workshops, Economic Models of Physician Behavior.* Chicago: University of Chicago Press.

Pear, Robert. 1993a. "Clinton's Health Care Plan: It's Still Big, but It's Farther Away." *The New York Times.* June 13.

———. 1993b. "Analysis Says Cost of Health Effort is Underestimated." *New York Times.* December 9.

———. 1993c. "Medicare to Stop Pushing Patients to Enter H.M.O.'s" *The New York Times.* December 27.

———. 1994a. "Behind the 'Policy Wonk Deal'," *New York Times.* February 10.

——— 1994b. "Medicare Paying Doctors 59% of Insurers' Rate, Panel Finds." *New York Times.* April 5.

Peterson, Peter G. 1993. *Facing Up, How to Rescue the Economy from Crushing Debt & Restore the American Dream.* New York: Simon and Schuster.

Pettengil, Julian. 1973. "The Financial Position of Private Community Hospitals, 1961–71." *Social Security Bulletin.* 36: (November) 3–19.

Plough, Alonzo L., Salem, Susanne R., Schwartz, Michael, Weller, John M., and Ferguson, C. William. 1984. "Case Mix in End-Stage Renal Disease—Difference between Patients in Hospital-Based and Free-Standing Treatment Facilities." *New England Journal of Medicine.* 310: (May 31) 1432–1436.

Pope, Gregory C., and Schneider, John E. 1992. "Trends in Physician Income." *Health Affairs*. 11: (Spring) 181–193.

Porter, Michael E. 1980. *Competitive Strategy, Techniques for Analyzing Industries and Competitors*. New York: The Free Press.

Prospective Payment Assessment Commission. 1993. *Medicare and the American Health Care System, Report to the Congress*. Washington, DC: PROPAC.

Reverby, Susan. 1979. "The Search for the Hospital Yardstick: Nursing and the Rationalization of Hospital Work." In *Health Care in America, Essays in Social History*. Reverby, Susan, and Rosner, David, ed. Philadelphia: Temple University Press.

Rice, Thomas, Brown, E. Richard, and Wyn, Roberta. 1993. "Holes in the Jackson Hole Approach to Health Care Reform." *Journal of American Medical Association*. 270: (Sept. 15) 1357–1362.

Rice, Thomas, and Thorpe, Kenneth E. 1993. "Income Related Cost Sharing in Health Insurance." *Health Affairs*. 12: (Spring) 21–39.

Robinson, James C., and Luft, Harold S. 1987. "Competition and the Cost of Hospital Care, 1972 to 1982." *Journal of American Medical Association* . 257: (June 19) 3241–3245.

———. 1988. "Competition, Regulation, and Hospital Costs, 1982–1986." *Journal of American Medical Association*. 260: (November 11) 2676–2681.

Roos, Nora P., Shapiro, Evelyn, and Tate, Robert. 1989. "Does a Small Minority of Elderly Account for a Majority of Health Expenditures? A Sixteen-year Perspective." *Milbank Quarterly*. 67: 347–369.

Rorem, C. Rufus. 1930. *The Public's Investment in Hospitals*. Chicago: University of Chicago Press.

Rosenbaum, David E. 1993. "America's Economic Outlaw: The U.S. Health Care System." *The New York Times*. October 26.

Rosenberg, Charles E. 1979. "The Origins of the American Hospital System." *Bulletin of the New York Academy of Medicine*. 55: (January) 10–21.

Rosenthal, Elisabeth. 1993. "Questions Raised on New Technique for Appendectomy." *New York Times*. September 14.

Rosner, David. 1979. "Business at the Bedside: Health Care in Brooklyn, 1890–1915." In *Health Care in America, Essays in Social History*. Reverby, Susan, and Rosner, David, ed. Philadelphia: Temple University Press.

Rublee, Dale A. 1989. "DataWatch: Medical Technology in Canada, Germany, and The United States." *Health Affairs*. 8: (Fall 1989) 178–181.

Rublee, Dale A., and Schneider, Markus. 1991. "International Health Spending: Comparisons with OECD." *Health Affairs*. 10: (Fall) 187–198.

Schieber, George J., Poullier, Jean-Pierre; and Greenwood, Leslie M. 1991. "Health Systems in Twenty-Four Countries." *Health Affairs*. 10: (Fall) 22–38.

———. 1992. "U.S. Health Expenditure Performance: An International Comparison and Data Update." *Health Care Financing Review*. 13: (Summer) 1–30.

Schroeder, Steven A., and Sandy, Lewis G. 1993. "Specialty Distribution of U.S. Physicians—The Invisible Driver of Health Care Costs." *New England Journal of Medicine*. 328 (April 1) 961–963.

Schur, Claudia L., and Taylor, Amy K. 1991. "Choice of Health Insurance and the Two-Worker Household." *Health Affairs.* 10: (Spring) 155–163.

Sigerist, Henry E. 1934. *American Medicine.* New York: W. W. Norton & Company.

Somers, Anne R., ed. 1971. *The Kaiser-Permanente Medical Care Program, A Symposium.* Oaklawn, CA: Kaiser Foundation Hospitals.

Somers, Herman Miles, and Somers, Anne Ramsey. 1961. *Doctors, Patients, and Health Insurance: The Organization and Financing of Medical Care.* Washington, DC: The Brookings Institution.

Soper, Nathaniel J., Brunt, L. Michael, and Kerbl, Kurt. 1994. "Medical Progress: Laparoscopic General Surgery." *New England Journal of Medicine.* 330: (February 10) 409–419.

Staff of the Committee on Finance of the United States Senate. 1970. *Medicare and Medicaid—Problems, Issues, and Alternatives.* Washington, DC: U.S. Government Printing Office.

Starr, Paul. 1982a. "Transformation in Defeat: The Changing Objectives of National Health Insurance, 1915–1980." *American Journal of Public Health.* 72: (January) 78–88.

———. 1982b. *The Social Transformation of American Medicine: The Rise of a Sovereign Profession and the Making of a Vast Industry.* New York: Basic Books, Inc.

Stevens, Rosemary. 1971. *American Medicine and the Public Interest.* New Haven: Yale University Press.

——— 1989. *In Sickness and in Wealth: American Hospitals in the Twentieth Century.* New York: Basic Books, Inc.

Swedlow, Alex, Johnson, Gregory, Smithline, Neil, and Milstein, Arnold. 1992. "Increased Costs and Rates of Use in the California Workers' Compensation System as a Result of Self-Referral by Physicians." *New England Journal of Medicine.* 327: (November 19) 1502–1506.

Tully, Shawn. 1992. "America's Painful Doctor Shortage." *Fortune.* 128: (November 16) 103–112.

U.S. Department of Commerce. 1992. *Statistical Abstract of the United States, 1992.* Washington, DC: U.S. Government Printing Office.

U.S. Department of Health, Education, and Welfare. 1972 and 1973. *Compendium of National Health Expenditures Data.* Washington, DC: Office of Research and Statistics, Social Security Administration.

———. 1976. *Health in America: 1776–1976.* Washington, DC: U.S. Public Health Service.

U.S. Senate Finance Committee Staff. 1970. *Medicare and Medicaid—Problems, Issues, and Alternatives: Report of the Staff.* Washington, DC: Government Printing Office.

Van Dyk, Frank. 1933. "A Group Hospital Insurance Plan." *Bulletin of the American Hospital Association.* 7: (January) 45–60.

Vogel, Morris J. 1980. *The Invention of the Modern Hospital: Boston 1870–1930.* Chicago: University of Chicago Press.

Waldo, Daniel R., Sonnefeld, Sally T., McKusick, David R., and Arnett, Ross H., III. 1989. "Health expenditures by age group, 1977 and 1987." *Health*

Care Financing Review. 10: (Summer) 111–121. And an Errata. *Health Care Financing Review.* 11: (Fall) 165–167.

Weeks, Lewis E., and Berman, Howard J. 1985. *Shapers of American Health Care Policy, An Oral History.* Ann Arbor, MI: Health Administration Press.

White, Jane H. 1993. "Understanding Clinton's Health Plan: Beyond Political Language." *Hospital Progress.* 74: (December) 14–18.

Winslow, Ron. 1993. "Big Firms Face Tough Health-Care Choice." *Wall Street Journal.* October 8.

Wolkstein, Irwin. 1968. "The Legislative History of Cost Reimbursement." In *Reimbursement Incentives for Hospital and Medical Care.* U.S. Department of Health, Education, and Welfare. Washington, DC: Social Security Administration.

Woolhandler, Steffie, Himmelstein, David U., and Lewontin, James P. 1993. "Administrative Costs in U.S. Hospitals." *New England Journal of Medicine.* 329: (August 5) 400–403.

Index

Blue Cross/Blue Shield (*continued*)
contracts, 63; national commission of, 64
Brown, E. Richard, 28, 121, 202n7

Califano, Joseph A., Jr., 91
California Public Employees Retirement System (CalPERS), 164
Canada, 130, 131, 132, 135, 136, 137, 138, 139, 140
Capital payments, in Medicare, 117
Capitation basis, 66, 70–71, 204n13
Carnegie Foundation, 28
Cartel(s), 47
Carter, Jimmy, 91, 95
Cataract surgery, 107
Catastrophically ill persons: as covered by federal programs, 178, 181; health care costs of, 177; insurance for, 197
Catholic Hospital Association, 46
Chandler, Alfred D., Jr., 38
Child Nutrition Act, 203n10
Clark, J. M., 150, 190
Clean Air Act, 203n10
Clean Water Restoration Act, 203n10
Cleveland Clinic Hospital, 40
Clinton, Bill, 1–2, 158–159. *See also* Clinton plan
Clinton, Hilary Rodman, 159
Clinton plan, 158–69; political constraints on, 166–69; summary of, 160–62
Cohn, Wilbur, 202–3n8
Commercialism, dangers of, in medicine, 12–13
Committee on Implication of For-Profit Enterprise in Health Care, 204n14
Committee on the Costs of Medical Care (CCMC), 45–46; minority report of, 46; report of, 48
Community Hospital-Clinic of Elk City, OK, 67
Community-wide rating system, 161, 165
Competition: among health insurers, 62–65; role of, 47
Competitive controls, 150
Comprehensive Health Planning

and Public Health Services Amendment, 203n10
Congressional Budget Office, 166–67
Consumer: apathy of re. health care, 124–27; as disenfranchised, 146; options of, under Clinton plan, 180–81; as passive, 121–27; as voters, 170–71
Consumer Price Index, 97
Cooper, Jim, 179
Copayment provisions, financing, 176
Cost-based reimbursement, 63
Cost sharing, income-related, 175
Cost shifting, 13, 89
Council on Medical Education, 28

Davis, Karen, 204n12
Davis, Michael, 50
Deductible payments, financing, 176
Dentistry and dentists: federal loans for, 70, 71; in Germany, 136
Department of Health, Education, and Welfare, 81
Department of Health and Human Services, 115
Diagnosis-related groups (DRGs), 115, 117; development of, 205n19
Diagnostic procedures: in hospital, 73–74; need to increase, 112
Disabled: under Clinton plan, 182; under Medicare, 91, 121
Disaggregation methodology, 134
Douglas, Paul, 203n9
Douglas amendment, 82
Drugs, hospital administered, 73, 135, 137; personal expenditures on, table, 78

Economic credentialing, 103
Economic Stabilization Program (ESP), 90–91, 97
Ellwood, Paul M., 163, 204n13, 205n22
Emergency Maternity and Infant Care Program, 200–201
Emergicenter, 102
Employees: under Clinton plan,

167; early retirement of, 182; lack of cost containment incentives for, 153–54
Employers: under Clinton plan, 160, 161–62, 179–80, 183–85, table, 184, 192; as health insurance administers, 52; as health insurance providers, 61, 153–54; and Kennedy plan, 166; obligations of, 198; options for, 127; risk avoidance by, 19–20; as self-insuring, 118; as sponsor of first dollar, free choice health insurance, 172
End-stage renal disease, 91, 100–102
Enthoven, Alain C., 163, 205n22
Entrepreneurship, 38–39. *See also* Physicians, as entrepreneurs
Experience rating, 65, 161

Federal government, role of in health care, 2–3. *See also* Clinton plan; Great Society; Medicare; Oligopsonist
Federal Home Owners Loan Corporation, 66
Fee-for-service basis, 65, 66, 119, 161, 191
Fee-splitting, 35
Feldstein, Martin, 84–85, 97, 176
Fetter, R. B., 205n19
Financing: health care costs, 174–80; national health care, 133–34; personal health services, 65–67
Finch, Robert, 88
First-dollar coverage, 83, 105, 146, 185. *See also* Free first dollar coverage; Last dollar coverage
Fishbein, Morris, 200n3
Fleming, Alexander, 57
Flexner, Abraham, report of, 27–29, 146, 199n1
Fogarty, John E., 60
Ford, Gerald, 91
Ford, Henry, 39
France, 130, 131, 132, 134, 135, 136, 139, 140
Freedom of choice, 65, 66, 79, 153
Free first (or low) dollar coverage, 170, 173. *See also* First dollar coverage; Last dollar coverage

Freestanding ambulatory surgery centers (FASCs), 107
Freshnock, Larry J., 103
Freymann, John Gordon, 57–58, 152
Fringe benefit(s): health care as, 55–57, 193
Fuchs, Victor, 138, 170, 185, 191, 194

Garfield, Sidney, 65
General practicioners (GPs): and open hospital staffing, 35; as outside health insurance payments, 77; retrocession of, 44–46; UK and U.S., 142
Germany, 130, 131, 132, 135, 136, 139, 140
GI bill, 68. *See also* Serviceman's Readjustment Act
Grandfathering, 28, 30, 146, 169
Great Depression, 42–43, 48; effect of on GPs, 144; and hospitals, 14, 109
Great Society program, 59
Gross domestic product (GDP), 130; allocation of, to health care, 7, 131–32
Group Health Association of Washington, 66, 67
Group Health Cooperative of Puget Sound, 66, 67
Group practices, increase in, 103

Hage, Jerald, 134
Hahn, James S., 138
Hanneman, Robert A., 134
Health care: access to, 9, 11; consumer apathy about price of, 124–27; consumer expenditures for, table,125, 126; developed nations' centralized budget for, 148–49; financing personal, 121–23, table, 122; as fringe benefit, 55–57; lack of organizational development in U.S.,16–17; seven developed nations (1960–1990), table, 131
Health care costs, 113–14; for catastrophically ill, 177; crisis in, 88–92; financing, 174–75; personal

Last-dollar coverage (*continued*)
172; as most appropriate for so-
cial insurance, 174
Lave, Judith, 59–60
Lave, Lester, 59–60
Law, Sylvia A., 202n7
Letsch, Suzanne W., 180, 181
Levit, Katharine R., 180, 181
Lewin-VHI study, 165
Lewontin, James P., 119
Licensure, 27, 29
Life expectancy, 86–87, 133
Life-styles, change in, 133
Lillie-Blanton, Marsha, 204n12
Lister, Joseph, 25
Long-term care, in Sweden, 135,
136
Low-dollar health insurance, 97, 99
Lowell, Francis, 26
Luft, Harold S., 203n11
Lyons, Barbara, 204n12

Magnetic resonance imaging (MRI)
units, 140
Mahoney, Florence, 60
Major medical benefits, 63
Managed care, 118, 173
Managed competition, 112, 163, 165
Marine Hospital Service, 202n6
Market failure: defined, 6; principal
source of, 153–56; symptoms of,
14–15
Markets, development of, 16–17
Markowitz, Gerald E., 28
Maternity admissions, rise in, 72–73
Mayo, Charles H., 40
Mayo, William J. (Will), 40, 70
Mayo, William W., 40
Mayo Clinic. *See* St. Mary's Hospital
McDermott, Jim, 166
Medicaid 2, 81; cutbacks in, 87–88;
eligibility for, 11; reduction in
state obligations for, 179
Medical bankruptcies, 89
Medical education: government sup-
port of, 4, 60, 61; as hospital-cen-
tered, 33
Medicare, 2; cost bulge of, 147; and
Clinton plan, 168–69, 178; cost ex-
plosion in, 83–86; disabled cov-
ered by, 121; federal loans for,

70; government expenditures for,
4; lack of cost containment incentives in, 154–55; legislative his-
tory of, 81–83; Part A, 81, 82,
116; Part B, 81, 82, 116, 125; pay-
roll tax for, 125; reimbursement
formula for, 203n9
Medigap policies, 121
Merchant Marine Hospital, 201n6
Mills, Wilbur, 81–82, 166
Milstein, Arnold, 112
Mitchell, Jean M., 112
Moloney, Thomas W., 142–43
Monheit, Alan C., 18, 178
Mortality rates, U. S., 1940–1980, ta-
ble, 86; U.S. in 20th century, ta-
ble, 57
Mullan, Fitzhugh, 204n12
Multihospital systems, 92–95;
chains, 94, 204n14, 205n17;
growth of, 111
"Mutual compulsion," 190

National Board of Medical Examin-
ers, 29
National Health Board, 161, 171,
187, 198
National health insurance (NHI), 2;
urgency of need for, 157–58
National Hospital Panel Survey,
117, 205n20
National Health Planning and Re-
sources Development Act of
1974, 91
National Institutes of Health, 58;
congressional appropriations for,
60; research grants of, 60, 145
National Labor Relations Board, 56
National Medical Care, 101
National Traffic and Motor Vehicle
Safety Act, 203n10
Neikirk, William, 186
Network HMOs, 119
New England Journal of Medicine, 12
New York Times, 5
Nixon, Richard, 88, 89
North American Free Trade Agree-
ment, 158
Nurse practitioners, 191
Nurse Training Act, 58